Miraculous
Health

Miraculous
Health

How to **heal** your **body** by **unleashing** the hidden **power** of your **mind**

DR. RICK LEVY
with Lou Aronica

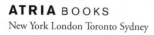
ATRIA BOOKS
New York London Toronto Sydney

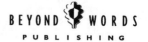
BEYOND WORDS
PUBLISHING

ATRIA BOOKS

A Division of Simon & Schuster, Inc.
1230 Avenue of the Americas
New York, NY 10020

BEYOND WORDS
PUBLISHING

20827 N.W. Cornell Road, Suite 500
Hillsboro, Oregon 97124-9808
503-531-8700 / 503-531-8773 fax
www.beyondword.com

The information contained in this book is intended to be educational and not for diagnosis, prescription, or treatment of any health disorder whatsoever. This information should not replace consultation with a competent healthcare professional. The content of the book is intended to be used as an adjunct to a rational and responsible healthcare program prescribed by a professional healthcare practitioner. The authors and publisher are in no way liable for any misuse of the material.

Editor: Julie Clayton-Knowles
Managing editor: Lindsay S. Brown
Copyeditor/proofreader: Henry Covey
Interior design: Sara E. Blum
Compositions: William H. Brunson Typography Services

First Atria Books/Beyond Words hardcover edition January 2008

ATRIA BOOKS and colophon are trademarks of Simon & Schuster, Inc.
Beyond Words Publishing is a division of Simon & Schuster, Inc.

For more information about special discounts for bulk purchases,
please contact Simon & Schuster Special Sales at 1-800-456-6798 or
business@simonandschuster.com.

Manufactured in the United States of America

10 9 8 7 6 5 4 3 2 1

Library of Congress Cataloging-in-Publication Data:

Levy, Rick.
    Miraculous health : how to heal your body by unleashing the hidden power of your mind /
by Rick Levy with Lou Aronica.
        p.   cm.
    1. Autogenic training—Therapeutic use.   2. Self-care, Health.   3. Mind and body.
    I. Aronica, Lou.   II. Title.
    RC499.A8L49   2008
    615.8'512—dc22
                                                                    2007025826

ISBN-13: 978-1-4391-0919-9

The corporate mission of Beyond Words Publishing, Inc.: *Inspire to Integrity*

TO

Paramahansa Yogananda

CONTENTS

Part Three: Treatment

Part Four: Supplemental Methods

Part Five: Preparing for the Rest of Your Life

ACKNOWLEDGEMENTS

This book would not have been possible without the hard work of a few visionary and talented people. First and foremost, my gratitude and devotion go to Lisa Tatum, MPM, MDiv, CH, my partner in work and life. Without her tireless efforts in helping me to write and her constant inspiration, this book would never have come into being. Similarly, I am forever indebted to my co-writer, Lou Aronica, whose knowledge of writing and publishing is only eclipsed by his patience. And thanks to my literary agent, Peter Miller, whose expertise made my dream become a reality.

My heartfelt thanks go to Linda Macek, LCSW, RN, for hours of painstaking work transcribing my numerous seminar talks, for her contribution to the chapter on cognitive reprogramming, and for conducting research in support of the glossary terms.

Thank you, Edward Boucher, my IT guru and friend, for bringing me into the twenty-first century technologically and for keeping me up and running in the world of electronic media against all the odds. My thanks also to Ellen Brown for helping me in myriad technical and practical ways and for her unwavering support. I want to recognize my intern Maria Thestrup (MA in psychology and doctoral candidate for a PhD in Clinical Psychology) for her research and editing which contributed to the chapter on cathartic and expressive techniques. My gratitude also to Dana Verkouteren, the gifted artist whose illustrations supplement the text.

Lastly, I want to thank Cynthia Black and Richard Cohn, my publishers, for their guidance and for taking a chance on me. And my dearest thanks to my daughters, Heather and Vicki, for all their love and support.

INTRODUCTION

"EVERY GREAT ADVANCE IN SCIENCE HAS ISSUED FROM
A NEW AUDACITY OF IMAGINATION."
—JOHN DEWEY

The field of mind-body science, the branch of medicine that looks at the mind's capacity to affect bodily health, is not new by a long shot—it is more than 4,000 years old—but the greatest advances have come about in the last twenty years, and it has been my special privilege and destiny to work on the cutting edge of this important frontier of medicine. Use of the mind to heal the body is not just a fascinating idea—it's hard science. Mind-body science has the ability to alleviate untold levels of human suffering, and in the not-too-distant future (when the best methods are widely available), it will be common practice.

I suppose I was uniquely prepared to expand the frontiers of mind-body medicine. I entered the profession of clinical psychology with the mind of a traditional hard-nosed scientist totally committed to improving the human condition, a family mantle I inherited from my father who was a world-class biochemist and brain researcher at the National Institutes of Health. After I earned my PhD in Clinical Psychology, I held a number of traditional leadership roles that included chairmanships of the Departments of Psychology at two state hospitals, Assistant Professor of Psychology at Frostburg University, and staff psychologist at St. Elizabeth's Hospital in Washington, D.C. Along the way, I led the National Hospital Privileges movement, which succeeded in winning hospital privileges for psychologists and ensured that patients in general hospitals would have access to psychological services. I also engineered the first credentialing standards for psychologists who practice in hospital settings. I was quite conservative—very "suit-and-tie"— devoted to the most rigorous scientific methods.

As far back as I can remember, I have been fascinated with human potential, the nature of thought, and the power of the human mind. As a child, I was quite gifted at mathematics, chemistry, and physics, which established in me a lifelong love for the hard sciences. In college, I began a thorough study of philosophy and world religion. By the time I hit graduate school, I had developed the heart of a religious mystic. In my private clinical practice, which began in 1976, I started to apply the objectivity of science to the unfettered vision of someone who believes in the limitlessness of human integrity and accomplishment. My approach to psychology not only included the application of rigorous psychological science and clinical method but also emphasized understanding the mind by exploring the worlds of philosophy, quantum physics, neurobiology, chemistry, religion, sociology, and anthropology.

It was through this unique synergy of knowledge that my private clinical practice became a living laboratory of human wonderment as I continued to discover and refine mind-body methods that delivered astounding results at every level of wellbeing. People with severe emotional and mental problems began to get better much more rapidly than previously thought possible, and their physical problems cleared up in the process—a woman with a serious case of depression was cured of her migraines; a man with an anxiety disorder was healed of Crohn's disease. As the list of breakthroughs kept growing, the preponderance of evidence became too great to deny—there was an obvious and profound connection between mental health and physical health and the mind-body methods I'd developed had a dramatic impact on both.

News of my success began to travel and so did I. I took my mind-body methods to five continents, to people of every culture, class, and age, from the world's international power-elite to the indigenous people of the Amazon and Africa. This vast experience demonstrated that the methods work universally well for all people and that anyone can apply them. In case after case, working with thousands of people from all walks of life who suffered from every kind of illness, I applied the knowledge and methods I'll show you in this book with staggering effect—rapid, significant, measurable gains in physical health and wellbeing, sometimes instantaneous and permanent after only one session.

By the late 1980s, I saw what the methods could do for people and realized their awesome implications for improving human wellbeing on a global scale. I became determined to get the methods out, even at the expense of my stature in the field of psychology (at that time, the clinical use of meditation, hypnosis, and biofield energy work were considered "fringe"). I used to joke in those days that I was "a suit-and-tie guy working in a tie-dye field," but as it turns out, I was merely ahead of the curve. In 2000, I testified as an expert witness for the White House Commission on Complementary and Alternative Medicine (CAM). The growing body of evidence for the effectiveness of mind-body medicine had finally pushed it into the medical mainstream.

Over three decades of clinical work, I have demonstrated that the power of the human mind is infinite, that every person possesses extraordinary nobility, and that life is a series of lessons designed to lead us into the direct experience of these two realities.

These are tall claims to be sure, but the methods speak for themselves. Their power cannot be denied. Try them and you will see. I'm not asking you to trust me; I'm asking you to trust your own experience and challenging you to have the audacity to imagine the limitless nature of your own power and greatness.

—Dr. Rick Levy

PRELUDE TO 1

A GLIMPSE INTO THE POWER OF THE MIND

If you have come to this book, it is probably because you are unwell. I am sorry that you are hurting, but we are going to start working on making you feel better immediately. I have spent my career helping people come into powerful levels of health and wholeness. Whether the issues that made you pick up this book are minor or major, or even life-threatening, roll up your sleeves and join me now on an adventure in self-healing. Together we will change your health and your life.

But first, we're going to start with something small. Think about something bothering you physically right now. Rate your level of pain, discomfort, or dysfunction on a scale of one to ten with ten being the worst pain imaginable ("It doesn't get any worse than this") and one being no pain at all ("I feel great"). Now, dim the lights, turn off the phone, sit back, close your eyes, and relax. I'm going to take you through a simple exercise that will show you that your mind is capable of exerting tremendous influence on your health and wellbeing.

Begin by monitoring your breath going in and out. Don't control it; just watch it go in and out on its own for a few breaths, putting all your attention on your breath without allowing any other thoughts to distract you. Next, begin silently counting backwards from ten to one. Count slowly, waiting about three seconds between each number. Now you're ready. Imagine the following scenario:

You go to a doctor for your health problem. He walks into the room and says, "Boy, are you in luck. We've just had a major breakthrough with this problem—a completely new way of treating it that we didn't have before. We're getting dramatic results! You couldn't have picked a better time to come in. You are so fortunate." The doctor then explains what this new breakthrough is. Maybe it's a new wonder drug, a new form of physical therapy or diet, or a new supplement or herbal medicine. Pick whatever feels best to you. The doctor tells you more about the drug and then says, "Follow this new regimen and you'll feel a lot better soon."

You leave the doctor's office feeling hopeful and energized. You jump right on the new therapy. Imagine yourself now taking the new medicine or supplement or going to physical therapy. Imagine that a little time goes by and you notice, "Hey, I am getting better. The doctor really knows what he's talking about. I'm really lucky to have gone in there when I did. This is really working."

Now imagine that you keep following the treatment routine. You find yourself feeling so great that you're actually feeling levels of joy you haven't felt in years and becoming optimistic about life again. You think, "I am so much better. I can't believe it."

Imagine a few weeks go by and you decide to go back to the doctor to see what he says. You make an appointment and the doctor checks you over. He smiles at you, puts his hand on your shoulder, and says, "You are doing great. You are well on your way to a complete recovery, speeding along like a track star. You're doing absolutely perfectly and I am so happy for you."

This is, of course, unbelievably good news for you and you feel fantastic. You're happy, you're well, and you're satisfied. It's like you've gotten a new lease on life.

Now, open your eyes and think about how you feel. How would you rate your pain, discomfort, or dysfunction? I'll bet you'll find it has improved. If it was a seven before, maybe it is a four or a three now.

You've just experienced the tiniest bit of what you will encounter over the course of this book. I designed this simple exercise to demonstrate that you can have an immediate effect on your physical health by using your mind as your greatest ally. Even if the improvement you feel now doesn't last, you've taken a glimpse into a remarkable new world, one in which your mind offers you the opportunity for miraculous health. I've been living in this world for nearly four decades now and can't wait to share it with you.

You already have everything inside of you that you require to permanently improve your physical wellbeing and feel great. All you need is someone to guide you along the way. I'm delighted to volunteer to serve as that guide.

Take my hand and hang on to your hat. I have miraculous things to show you.

CHAPTER 1

The Story Behind the Story

I f I asked you to tell me your life story right now, what would you say? In all likelihood, you'd give me details about where you were born, how you grew up, the house you moved to when you were twelve, where you went to school, what you do for a living, and so on. Maybe you'd tell me about your first love or your first heartbreak.

But would you tell me about the signal events that made you who you are now? Probably not, because you're most likely not even conscious of these. Most people aren't. For example, consider one of my patients from 1997.

Erin, a successful healthcare professional, flew in to see me from St. Paul. She'd married late in life, and now thirty-nine, was trying to have a child. She had suffered three miscarriages in the past eighteen months—one of which was very late term—and understandably, she was extremely upset. Her most significant medical problem was that she had an inverted uterus, a congenital condition. Several gynecologists told her it would be nearly impossible to carry a child to term because of this.

During our first meeting, I asked her to tell me more about herself. Erin was born into a prominent family, but her mother died tragically when Erin was eleven. This event plunged the entire family into despair, disarray, and ultimately, for Erin, poverty. In the years that followed, Erin struggled with depression and a major back injury while doing everything she could to make her life successful. She put herself through two graduate degrees, visited a psychotherapist regularly, pursued philosophical and religious studies, and traveled the world. Now she was at a crucial turning point, desperately wanting to have a child and to build her own healthy, loving family. From her perspective, doing so was the most important goal in the world.

That was her history.

Her *story behind the story* was another matter.

As Erin spoke to me, I knew something more was going on than what I could learn from the bullet points of her life. *Everyone* has a deeper story that goes beyond the mere events in their lives. This deeper story has a tremendous effect on us, one that is so much more intense than what we normally associate with our life stories. Yet, most of us remain unaware of a deeper story because we can't figure out a way to reach it—because we don't even know it exists.

To get to Erin's *story behind the story*, I guided her into a hypnotic state and asked her to go to the place in her mind where she would find the knowledge she needed to get well. She went to the day of her mother's death and experienced those moments as though she was there again. She told me who was there with her, what people were saying, and what she felt.

Suddenly, she gasped and said, "Pregnancy leads to death." I asked her to elaborate on this, and she told me her mother was seven months pregnant when she died. Since Erin was at the impressionable age of eleven, she linked the two events in her mind. She intertwined pregnancy and death and secreted this distorted "belief" in her subconscious from that day forward. Now this distortion was fueling her miscarriages because the subconscious mind has the important job of preserving our physical survival.

As soon as Erin found this distortion under hypnosis, she released it quickly (we'll discuss how this happens later in the book), breaking the link between these two concepts. At this point, the unfortunate connection she'd created between pregnancy and death could no longer do her physical harm. She'd found the part of her story that was preventing her from bringing a child into the world—and she rejected it.

Within three months, Erin called me to say she was pregnant. Despite her inverted uterus, she carried her son to term and started the family she desperately wanted. And in so doing, she changed her story.

THE INEXTRICABLE CONNECTION BETWEEN THE MIND AND THE BODY

Since you are reading this book, you are probably among the large percentage of people with health problems who have found that traditional medicine fails to deliver the quality of life they desire. Because of my expertise, many people who feel this way come to me for help—often after their physicians have told them that chronic pain, depression, anxiety, dysfunction, disability, or even the specter of death are unavoidable.

Most of these people come to me in a state of despair for understandable reasons. They believe their illness has caused this despair. That is usually when I introduce them to the first lesson in mind-body science. "If that's what you think," I say, "you've put the cart before the horse." Most people who feel bad physically got that way and stay that way because, whether they know it or not, they were not satisfied with their lives to begin with. They were living stories that made them deeply unhappy in ways they could barely understand.

You might not believe this. You might point to a family history of diabetes, a congenital heart disorder, a fractured back in a car accident, or the degradations of twenty years of smoking. "These are the reasons I'm sick," you'll say, "not some vague concept about some story I'm living out." If you feel this way now, I ask you to stick with me because I'll prove that you're not seeing things as clearly as you think you're seeing them. All of the issues above might be relevant to the onset of suffering, but they are not the only causes of illness.

More importantly, they are not keys to a cure. The key comes in a simple but powerful revelation that I will repeat often in this book: disease in the body starts with dis-ease in the mind. Any health issue you have corresponds directly to some level of distortion in your mind. Therefore, to set free the hidden power of the mind for healing, you need to discover that distortion. You need to get to the *story behind the story*.

Every one of us is living a unique, epic journey, an adventure in self-discovery and self-knowledge. The plots vary widely, leading us through the extremes of poverty and wealth, triumph and despair, love and loneliness, strength and weakness, illness and health, grace and shame. Everyone's lessons in life are different. However, everyone's story has the possibility of a noble outcome, and everyone's potential is truly unlimited if they are willing to live their own story deeply and honestly.

Living outside your story—failing to learn the lessons life is trying to teach you or misunderstanding or repressing your experience—is the root cause of pain and suffering. When I say this, I do not mean to imply that you are purposely ignoring your life lessons. We human beings tend to repress any experience we find painful, terrifying, difficult, shameful, or otherwise challenging, so we can move on in life. We do it subconsciously because we have to in order to maintain our stability and forward momentum—we have jobs, school, children, and other important responsibilities that need our attention. So we sacrifice our personal needs. Unfortunately, powerful feelings, thoughts, and desires that are repressed or "set aside" in this manner remain in the subconscious mind where they sabotage our psychological, physical, and spiritual wellbeing.

The good news is, if you can identify your story and live it out authentically, you can unleash miraculous mental power and attain great health, peace, and joy. Your age, station in life, race, culture, gender, or how much suffering you've had to endure doesn't matter.

It really is that simple.

However, *getting* to your *story behind the story* is not so simple. Because the human mind is a complex machine, you'll need some tools to get there. I will provide those tools in this book. These tools will help you get in touch with parts of your mind you've had little or no access to in the past. They will help you understand the themes, long-buried memories, and unacknowledged lessons you learned from others that have had a profound effect on your life. They will help you see the life you've lived in ways you've never seen before and help you decide which parts of that life you want to keep and which parts you want to change.

In short, these tools will change everything, for the better.

Most people are only aware of their conscious thoughts, beliefs, and attitudes, but conscious awareness is the smallest, weakest part of the mind. The subconscious mind is much larger and more powerful, and you are living out much of your story there. A rule of thumb we use in the field of clinical hypnosis is that the subconscious mind is two to two and a half times the size and power of the conscious mind.

In addition, there is the vastness of the super-conscious mind—what people commonly call the "soul" or "spirit" (we'll discuss this at length later). Every human being possesses super-conscious awareness, and it is infinite in power. Some of your story is being lived out there in the form of your highest aspirations, your search for meaning, your yearning for what is sacred, and your knowledge that there is so much more to life. In a recent Gallup poll, 82 percent of people in the United States professed a belief in God and another 13 percent professed a belief in a higher power. When you experience the *story behind your story*, you'll encounter revelations that, if you are religious, you will see as coming from God. If you are a scientific humanist, you'll see these revelations as coming from deep within yourself. No particular point of view is needed to succeed with my methods. All of us, independent of belief, are capable of tapping the tremendous healing power contained in the super-conscious mind.

For each of us, the resources in the subconscious and super-conscious constitute a limitless storehouse of mental energy that has the ability to heal the body and mind, address the challenges of day-to-day living, and sustain an extraordinary life of fulfillment and joy. As I have done for thousands of my patients, I will show you how to tap into the knowledge and power that are secreted away in your mind. It will give you the ability to live life large and my guess is that once you have a taste of it, you're going to want to explore it more deeply.

WHAT DO YOU BELIEVE?

"You are what you believe." Most people would agree with that statement. What we believe determines how we see ourselves, how we relate to our bodies, how we relate to others and to the world, and ultimately how we feel, but do you really know what you believe at a deep, subconscious level? Most people—with the rare exception of those who have pursued a disciplined effort at self-knowledge—are unaware of their own true beliefs.

There are two reasons why. The first is that you've filed the vast majority of your experience (memory) and thoughts (beliefs) away in your subconscious (often long ago, when you were a child), and you can't access them through ordinary means. Think of Erin, who was shocked to discover that she believed pregnancy would lead to death. Erin had no idea she felt that way, but this subconscious belief led to her recurrent miscarriages.

The second reason is that what we believe may or may not be an accurate reflection of reality. What we believe is simply a product of our experience and education, our conditioned habits of thought, our general level of awareness, and the workings of our brains—all of which are highly subjective. One of the first things I do for my patients who have serious health problems is to challenge what they hold dear. I help them deconstruct and then reconstruct their belief systems. This is a necessary first step toward going beyond one's limited reality. You will learn how to do this for yourself in this book. It requires some effort but it is well within your reach.

Everyone thinks they are living in the "real world," but this is rarely true. Over the course of this book, you will learn that you are living in a box determined by your brain and your mental conditioning, and you will discover the tools to free yourself from the limitations of that box.

About five years ago, I was sitting in a beautifully renovated playhouse in Greensboro, North Carolina, watching my daughter play the lead role of Maria in *West Side Story*. It was a father's dream come true. She was fantastic, seemingly right there in Spanish Harlem, standing on a fire escape on the second floor of a tenement building. At intermission, though, I walked up to the stage—a set design, painted on a wall just a few inches thick. From this perspective, it was obvious the stage was nothing but an illusion. When I went back to my seat for the second act, however, the drama and music mesmerized me again; I could swear it was real.

The "real world" is such an illusion. Look at what you "see" in the room around you. Now consider how other species would regard the same thing. A fly simultaneously sees dozens of pictures of its immediate environment. Bats navigate using radar, an entirely different system from ours. A dog doesn't see color but can smell, hear, and feel things that human beings do not. As part of its own survival strategy, each species constructs its own world of sensory impressions out of the energies around it. Whose worldview is more accurate? During the Asian tsunami crisis in December 2004, news agencies reported a compelling phenomenon: the wild and domestic animals in Sumatra fled to the mountains in the hours before the tsunami struck. They knew, through their ability to tune in to electromagnetic energy patterns, about the oncoming devastation. If only the human inhabitants of Sumatra could have known how to do the same thing.

Of course, human beings can tune in to electromagnetic energies, and we have the mental power to manage this energy to some degree. You will need this skill in order to heal yourself, and I will teach it to you in this book.

The world you live in is a reflection of the map of your own neurology and your thoughts and beliefs, stimulated by electromagnetic energy. You are neither experiencing an objective reality (though you think you are) nor interpreting it objectively. Like the backdrop in my daughter's play, what you're sensing is just a stage set.

How well do you perceive the stage set for your own life story? Probably not as well as you think. Consider the mechanism by which we "see" an object—a new car, for example. A light wave from the car hits a receptor nerve cell in your eye. At the same time, electrical energy is running from your brain into this nerve cell. The two currents of energy meet and an electrical signal goes to the brain. Then, the mind has to perceive or interpret the signal that's been received by the brain. That's where your thoughts, beliefs, and general level of awareness come in.

At any step along this process, there is room for substantial error. If you have too little energy in your nerves, as would be the case if you have a neurological problem, you won't actually "see" correctly because insufficient electrical current is going to the brain. Or perhaps this is the first "car" you've ever seen, in which case you still won't "see" objectively because your thoughts and beliefs provide no model for interpreting the signal.

I saw this phenomenon in 1998 when working with the Shuar, a tribe of headhunters in Amazonian Ecuador. Most of the Shuar had never seen a white person or any form of modern technology. A close colleague of mine on that expedition had left the Shuar village years before to go to the "big city" to get an education. She described her experience the first time she encountered a door. Since the Shuar don't have doors on their grass huts, she stood for a long time in front of the door, pushing on it, growing increasingly frustrated. She did not "see" the doorknob because her mind had no basis for perceiving what she was looking at.

Before you say, "Well, those were a primitive people . . . *I'm* not unaware of things in my environment," think again. The human brain receives more than eleven million sensory inputs every minute, of which most people are aware of a scant 2 percent. Each of us lives in a box of our own creation. As it turns out, it's a very small box indeed, but I can help you make yours much, much larger. In fact, I can teach you how to get out of the limitations of your box altogether.

THE NEED TO REEVALUATE YOUR CONSTRUCT OF WHAT IS "REAL"

The reason you should learn to deconstruct your ideas about what is "real" (as you will be able to do via the tools in this book) is that the boxes we create and live in can become prisons that threaten our physical health and wellbeing. Just as the world you thought was real is only a box of your own creation, the "you" that you presently experience is not a reflection of reality either. Nor is it fixed. We human beings are also composed of energy: from the electrons, neutrons, and protons, which form the building blocks of cellular structure in the body, to the electric impulses that govern the human heartbeat and drive our senses. We are not merely biological beings composed of chemicals and chemical processes; we are also biophysical beings composed of energy.

Similarly, human thought and feeling exist as subtle energy. An electroencephalograph (EEG) measures a patient's brain activity in the form of energy waves whose amplitude and frequency correlate with various states of consciousness (waking or sleeping, anxious or calm, reasoning or imagining, for example). This illustration leads me to the most essential tenet of mind-body medicine: human thought and feeling translate instantaneously into biophysical change (in this case, altered brainwave patterns). According to a recent survey by the American Psychological Association, 80 percent of Americans believe you cannot have good physical health unless you have good mental health. They are entirely correct. Every physical illness, even those caused by injury, has a root cause in the mind. As I said earlier, every disease in the body begins with dis-ease.

Therefore, if your body is ailing, you will be able to find a related ailment or distortion in your thinking (most of which goes on at the subconscious and super-conscious levels within the mind). It is critically important for people with a physical illness to be able to access the content of their thought at all levels (conscious, subconscious, and super-conscious) as a means to healing. In the chapters that follow, I will teach you how to feel the energies in your body and use deep levels of awareness to access your thoughts so you can direct those energies, shift what is going on in your bodily tissues, and achieve self-healing.

The power of these techniques (energy work combined with increased access to the power in your subconscious and super-conscious minds—the techniques you will learn in this book) is often miraculous. I saw this with a patient of mine named John, who I met at a conference on alternative healthcare in Fredericksburg in 1996. He was fifty-one years old and had suffered from juvenile diabetes for most of his life. By the time I met him, he was nearly blind. The sight in one eye was functioning at 40 percent, and the other eye was functioning at only 15 percent. I began to do energy therapy on his eyes while guiding John into a hypnotic state (a heightened state of inner awareness that allows a person full access to the content of the mind) and asked him to talk to me about what he did not want to see in his life.

John might well have said, "What do you mean 'what I don't want to see?' I have diabetes!" Instead, he spoke with deep feeling about the fact that he had no surviving relatives and about his longstanding fear that he would end up homeless and destitute. He explored this at length and began to realize he had the resources to avoid this dismal future. In spite of the deaths in his family, he had enough money to get by and people who cared for him. As he realized this, he naturally let go of his distorted beliefs, and the vision in both eyes began to improve noticeably. A week later, an eye exam showed that the eye operating at 15 percent before had risen to 80 percent, while the eye operating at 40 percent was now functioning at 85 percent.

John's history was that he had juvenile diabetes and was losing his sight. The root cause of his declining vision, though, was that he'd seen so much tragedy in his life and gotten to the point where he didn't want to see any more. John's mind had built up the distorted belief that life was a series of disasters and that the future only brought more heartache. His *story behind the story* was that John subconsciously did not want to "see" himself become alone and abandoned. Therefore, his mind systematically shut off his sight.

When he let go of his distorted beliefs—when he made the decision to change his story—he was free to look at the world around him again. The tools in this book will allow you to do something equally dramatic if that's what you want.

Repeatedly, over my thirty years of clinical work, I have seen that when we get to our *story behind the story*, amazing healing occurs. John could have written his blindness off to juvenile diabetes. Erin could have assumed her physical problems meant the death of her dream to have a child. They, however, were willing to look deeper than the physical symptoms, explore their minds for distorted beliefs, release those beliefs, and revise their stories in a way that dramatically improved their health—and led them to richer and happier lives at the same time.

It's your turn now. Once you are able to access your *story behind the story* you will be amazed at how much better you will feel both physically and emotionally. You will rid yourself of the hidden pain and delusion that is sabotaging your body. You will reject the parts of your story that encumber you. You will celebrate the noblest parts of your story—parts you might not have realized were yours at all—and decide to make the rest of your story something to celebrate as well. If you truly want to, you can employ the tools in this book to become the best person you can possibly be. They can even lead you to the heights of human greatness.

You have no idea how powerful you are. This is true even if you already think you are powerful. Think of someone who has overcome the odds and demonstrated tremendous strength and character. Lance Armstrong, seven-time winner of the Tour de France, overcame testicular cancer, which should have killed him, then started a worldwide movement for cancer awareness and research. You can be that powerful.

What is the difference between Lance Armstrong and you? Nothing! Except that he knows how powerful he can be, and you probably do not know how powerful you are. Like Lance Armstrong, you can achieve any noble goal you set your heart to.

People like Lance Armstrong refuse to buy in to two big lies that permeate our culture and hold people back. The first lie is, "Hey, achieving your dreams and having a wonderful life really isn't possible." The second is, "Oh yeah, it's possible all right; it's possible for Lance Armstrong but not for me. I'm just not good enough." I can tell you that, based on three decades of clinical work with people from every station of life, nothing is further from the truth. It's going to take some work—nothing this magnificent comes without effort—but if you endeavor to learn the tools in this book, you'll experience a wonderful payoff. You'll discover your *story behind the story*, bask in the limitless power of your mind, feel better than you've felt in years, and swim in the extravagant joy that is every human being's birthright.

It's all waiting for you.

BEFORE YOU MOVE AHEAD

I always describe my methods as "Integrative Medicine," meaning they are ideally used together with conventional healthcare (medical care provided by a physician, nurse practitioner, or properly credentialed mental health professional). Please be wise. Seek conventional medical treatment in response to your healthcare needs and use the methods in this book to magnify your health and wellbeing. If you have no access to appropriate medical care, then by all means, use the methods in this book to heal yourself. The methods are very powerful, in many cases powerful enough to stand alone as a cure. However, they are not designed to replace conventional medical care and should not be used in exchange for common sense. Please be smart. Use *all* the tools available to you, and you will be well.

PART ONE

SKILL BUILDING

PRELUDE TO 2

THOUGHT DIRECTS THE ENERGY INSIDE OF YOU

This simple exercise will get you "in touch" with the way your mind can affect the energy in your body. First, notice how both of your hands feel right now. Perhaps there is a bit of tingling in your fingertips and some warmth in the center of your palms. Both hands probably feel about the same. Now, prepare for this exercise in the same way that you prepared for the exercise at the start of chapter 1, by relaxing and focusing the mind. Turn off the phone, sit back, close your eyes, and relax. Start to monitor your breath going in and out. Don't force the breath or time it in any way, just watch it go in and out on its own for a few breaths, concentrating exclusively on the flow. Next, begin silently counting backwards from ten to one. Count slowly, waiting about three seconds between each number. Now you're ready to begin. Take four to five minutes to imagine the following:

You take your left hand and plunge it into a bucket of extremely cold water—and I mean cold, really cold. Imagine a bucket of cold water into which someone is continually adding trays of ice cubes. It's excruciatingly cold. After a few moments, you notice your fingers feel numb and then the feeling gets more intense. It starts at the tips of the fingers, moves up through the knuckles, to the palm, and then all the way through your hand. Now your whole hand is getting unbelievably cold. You start to shiver as the cold works up your arm and into your body. You are thinking, "I have to get my hand out of this water."

Now shift your attention to the right hand. Imagine putting your right hand into a bucket of extremely hot water. As your hand goes in the bucket, your immediate thought is, "I'm not sure I can even keep my hand in this thing!" And the water keeps getting hotter. Imagine the hottest tap water is in the bucket to begin with and that someone is using a teakettle full of boiling water to refresh the bucket at intervals. Now it's so hot it feels like it is burning the skin off your hand. Still, you leave your hand in the bucket. The heat is almost unbearable. You can feel it crawling up your fingers, all the way back to your palm. Your palm is even starting to swell. You feel like your hand and fingers are cooking. You can feel your brow begin to perspire. Finally, you can't stand it anymore. You have to get your hand out of the hot water, and you yank it out.

Now, stop imagining, open your eyes, and notice how different your hands feel. Each hand feels different, doesn't it? This change resulted exclusively from your mind's ability to effect the energetic sensations in your hands.

Your thoughts direct the energy in your body, a subject we take up in the next chapter.

Soon you will be in touch with the energetic sensations in your body, and more importantly, you will be able to put them to work to improve your health and the health of those around you.

CHAPTER 2

FEELING ENERGY

B efore you learn to use the tremendous power within you to heal yourself and others, you need to learn to use a number of basic tools. Each
of these tools will immediately provide you with a bit of healing power. As
you get better at using each of them and then begin to use them in concert
with one another, their value grows exponentially. If you start working with
these tools today and spend some time working on them every day thereafter, you should feel profound changes within a few short weeks.

There are two keys to gaining the most from part 1 of this book. The
first is patience. You likely came to this book because you or someone
important to you is unwell. You or someone you love might even be in considerable pain. I know it will be tempting for you to try to jump-start the
results here—to rush through the process and jump to the middle to "turn
this thing on" the way you might with a new computer or piece of audio
equipment. Try to avoid this temptation. As I said in the last chapter, you're
going to need to commit some time and effort to gain the wonders available
to you. If you try to jump ahead too quickly, you won't generate the power
you need. Sorry, but there's no way around this. All I can promise is that if
you dedicate yourself, your patience will be rewarded.

You'll need to practice the techniques described in these opening chapters
for several days before you're ready to move on to the remainder of the book.
The time you spend building these skills now will make a huge difference in

the level of healing power you'll be able to generate. A bit of patience and dedication now will deliver a lifetime of extraordinary dividends.

The second key is open-mindedness. The scientific mind is not a closed mind. I always tell my clients, "Hey, you don't have to believe me up front, but be a good scientist and a good empirical observer—try the methods, observe what happens, and go with your own experience." As you work through the stages of this book, keep an open mind and pay attention to what happens. If some of this fails to "make sense" at first or doesn't fit with some of your established notions, that's a good thing. It means your worldview is opening up, along with endless possibilities.

I'm not asking you to trust me; I'm asking you to trust yourself.

WE ARE ALL ENERGY

In 1998, I was a presenter at a conference on alternative medicine in Washington, D.C. After my seminar on how to manipulate bio-electromagnetic (BioEM) energy fields to heal physical problems, I invited volunteers to come to the dais from the audience. Up walked a woman, laboring badly with the aid of a tripod cane. She had been a dancer in her youth and her knees had worn down on her completely. Knee surgeries had done little to help. For about fifteen minutes, I used biofield therapy techniques (more on this in a few pages), giving powerful doses of healing energy to her injured knees.

What happened next was like something from an old movie. The woman stood, smiled broadly—and she began to dance about, right there on the stage, ecstatic with her newfound health. She left the auditorium without the use of her cane to huge applause.

Five years later, I was sitting in the front row at another conference, waiting for my turn as speaker. This same woman took the seat next to me. "You don't remember me, do you?" she said smiling. Terribly abashed, I had to confess that I recognized her but couldn't remember her name—a professional hazard when you see so many people for brief encounters. She reintroduced herself and told me that she registered for this conference because she knew I'd be speaking and wanted to thank me. She went on to explain that after I healed her knees, she embarked on a three-month tour of Europe, followed by three weeks in Australia. Her life had been one great adventure since she regained the use of her legs. She felt as spry today as she did those moments after leaving the stage.

That's what's possible when you learn to feel BioEM energy and use it to promote healing. You can do this yourself if you take the time to learn and practice the techniques to come.

Like the world we live in, we are composed of atomic and subatomic particles, space, and electromagnetic energy fields. You are made of energy. Thought directs energy, and as a result, it directs the structure and functioning of your body, your relationships with others, and your overall wellbeing.

Energy flowing throughout the body creates BioEM energy fields in and around the body. The composition, size, balance, and movement of these fields correlate with various states of physical, mental, and spiritual health, and you will learn in this book how to interpret this information.

A long-established fact of Western science is that the body is composed of BioEM energy and that one can use this energy for healing. The first BioEM field documented in the West was the field of the heart, discovered by Willem Einthoven a century ago. His research led to the electrocardiogram and won him the Nobel in 1924. A quarter of a century later, Hans Berger measured the electrical fields of the brain, resulting in the discipline of electroencephalography. Today, conventional medicine uses energy to restructure damaged nerves, repair aneurisms, destroy cancer cells, and break up bone-based scar tissue. For example, Functional Electrical Stimulation (FES) is a technique that uses low-level electrical currents to reactivate nerves in the arms and legs of people who suffer paralysis resulting from spinal cord injury, head injury, or stroke.

Biofield therapy—using simple *mentalistic* means to manipulate BioEM energies—is much more powerful and versatile than conventional energy medicine. It can often stand alone as a cure. I have had countless experiences like the one earlier in this chapter of complete and instantaneous healing using only biofield therapy.

Biofield therapy can rapidly decrease discomfort. In many cases, it can get rid of pain completely. Repeated applications of biofield therapy can reduce inflammation, heal problems that have been resistant to traditional medical approaches, and heal even the most stubborn, life-threatening conditions. Think about what this means to you. If you invest some of yourself now in learning the technique, you will have a tremendous ability to make yourself and others feel dramatically better. If you or someone you love is in any level of physical distress, you have within your mind the ability to help heal it. With practice using my methods, you will even perceive physical problems before you see any symptoms—and, as every doctor knows, the earlier the intervention, the better the chance for a cure. These methods are that potent. I will provide you with all the tools you need, but first, let me give you just a little more background.

THOUGHT AS ENERGY

Thought exists as subtle electromagnetic energy. In contrast to outdated psychological theories that assumed your thoughts stayed within the privacy of your own head, science long ago proved that thoughts permeate your body and radiate out into the world in the form of electromagnetic energy waves. When these waves come in contact with another energy field (whether it is the field surrounding your own heart, the field of another person, or the field connected to a place or set of circumstances), they have a deciding influence on what is happening. Simply put, what you think determines your health, future, and ability to influence the wellbeing of others.

Dr. Masaru Emoto, author of *The Hidden Messages in Water* and other books on the subject, has demonstrated conclusively that human thought changes the subatomic composition of water crystals. Different thoughts, such as "hate" or "love," create changes in water crystals visible through a microscope. In a group experiment conducted in Washington, D.C., in 1993, researchers collaborated with the D.C. Metropolitan Police Department in an attempt to reduce violent crime. Four thousand people agreed to meditate on the problem—that's four thousand personal BioEM fields focusing their mental energy on a large, complex set of energies associated with criminal tendencies, pockets of social oppression, and so on. The result: violent crime in Washington, D.C., dropped by an unprecedented 25 percent in the ensuing days.

In subsequent chapters, I will teach you how to employ different ways of thinking to direct BioEM energies to improve the wellbeing of you and your loved ones. For now, it is important for you to realize that what you're thinking will help determine your experience. As you work through the exercises at the end of this chapter, then, allow yourself to think big. Realize that you have extraordinary levels of power in your mind. Let yourself use these powers. Open yourself to the incredible potential that exists inside you. You'll be astounded with the results.

STRENGTHENING THE BODY'S OWN INTELLIGENCE

Eastern medicine has long understood what we have rediscovered only in the last decade of research in mind-body medicine: your body has an inherent intelligence; it "knows" how to heal and sustain itself. This is the foundation of all of Eastern medicine. When you cut yourself, your body knows how to heal the cut. Why, then, do some cuts heal more slowly than others? A knee scrape might take a few days to heal one time and a few weeks another. This happens because of differing levels of energy in your body. If your body is physically exhausted from stress or lack of sleep, for instance, healing takes more time. Biofield therapy supercharges your body and allows it to do more of what its natural intelligence would have it do.

Anyone can learn how to do biofield therapy. If you commit yourself to practicing the techniques in this book, you'll be very good at it very quickly. The first step is learning how to feel the body's energies and move them. Once you begin to develop this skill, you can benefit from it immediately and be well on your way to doing this like a pro in a short time.

EXERCISE 1: CREATING THE ENERGY BUBBLE

The first step in gaining awareness and a certain level of influence over your BioEM energy fields is to learn to feel them. Eventually, you will be able to do this with your entire body, but we're going to begin with the basics: feeling energy with your hands.

Put your hands as close together as you can get them without touching, perhaps one-quarter of an inch or so apart. They should be out in front of you and perpendicular to the floor (see fig. 1).

Do you feel anything? Pay careful attention to this sensation and how it changes in the next stages.

Next, take one hand and while keeping it parallel to the other hand, lift it above the other. Do this very slowly; it should take about fifteen seconds for one hand to be completely above the other. Pay close attention to how

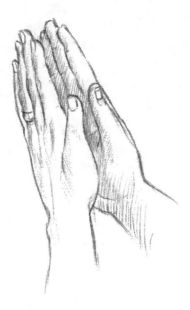

FIGURE 1

your hands feel while they are moving and when they stop. In what ways is it different from what you felt when your hands were together?

Now, even more slowly, move the hand back down again. Notice what feelings come to you in the palms of your hands. You are likely to feel the following:

- A sense of warmth between your hands. This is because of radiant energy traveling between them.
- Tingling in your palms or in the tips of your fingers. This is because there are fine energy centers in the palms and fingertips that are especially sensitive to energy.
- A feeling like thin foam rubber between your hands: a sense of resistance and then a sense of attraction between the hands. This is because you are compressing the electromagnetic fields that emanate from each hand, and when your hands get very close together, these fields penetrate each other.

Once you have a strong sense of what you're feeling, you can learn how to infuse the body with energy and direct this energy effectively. Move your hands about a foot from your body with one palm open and facing to the side and a finger from the opposite hand pointing to that palm (see fig. 2).

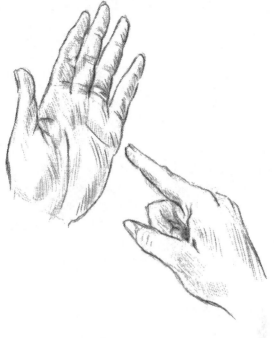

FIGURE 2

Move the pointed finger to the center of your palm slowly and feel the energies coming off the tip of the finger. When the pointed finger is about a half of an inch from your palm, slowly start moving that finger parallel to the floor away from you. What do you feel? Reverse direction and see if you feel something different. Create a circle or write a letter or number. Most people can sense the trace outline. You might even feel the energy penetrate all the way through and cause tingling on the back of your hand.

The next step is to develop a greater awareness of what is going on between your hands. The best way to do this is to "play patty-cake." Slowly move your hands out from one another—maybe an inch apart. Then very slowly move them closer again without touching. Do this a few times and then extend the distance—first two inches, then four, then six. You should notice a sense of "squishiness." The foam rubber feeling has expanded and seems malleable. This squishiness between your hands is an energy bubble and is an extremely powerful healing device.

Now create the bubble and make it wide enough to put your knee between your hands. Hold the bubble there for fifteen seconds or so. What do you feel? Most people feel a sense of warmth or maybe even some tingling in the knee. This is because you are feeding your knee with energy. If you can easily reach a part of your body where you have some pain, place the bubble there and hold it for five minutes or so. This might seem like a long time to you, but it will take that long or longer at the beginning.

What do you feel? The pain should subside, at least a little. This is because the energy you're contributing is working with your body's natural intelligence to affect healing. This is the tiniest hint of what you'll be able to do once you've practiced more. You'll be stunned at what you'll be able to do a few weeks from now.

If you are paralyzed or otherwise immobilized by illness and cannot apply this technique (or some of the other biofield energy techniques in this chapter), you have other options available to you. First, you can have someone else learn the methods in this chapter and apply them to your body. Even if your companion is new to the technique(s), you will feel some positive results. You can also effectively use exercise 4 in this chapter to great effect, as it requires no movement at all. In addition, there are other methods in the book (such as those in chapters 11 and 12) you can use to increase the amount of energy available to a diseased or injured part of your body, methods that involve only the power of your mind, without any physical movement required.

EXERCISE 2: USING THE BUBBLE TO MOVE ENERGY

At this point, a partner is useful to work with. If you do not feel comfortable asking someone you know to work with you on these skills, you can consider going to my website, www.miraculoushealthbook.com. There, you can post a need for a partner on our bulletin board.

If possible, try using the energy bubble you've learned to create on your partner. Perhaps she has a headache. Ask her to grade the pain from this headache on a scale of one to ten, with ten being the worst pain she can imagine and one being no pain at all. Then create the energy bubble using the "patty-cake" method and hold your hands up to your partner's head, one in front and one in back. Leave your hands there for several minutes and let the energy flow from your hands. Do not touch your partner's head. Try visualizing energy flowing from your hands into your partner's head to increase the amount of energy you are moving and its healing effect (remember, thought directs energy). If you do this, your partner should feel a significant drop in pain. In five minutes time, her pain might be half of what it was.

While you hold your hands there, notice what you feel. Most people notice that one hand feels like it has more energy flowing through it. This is your stronger healing hand. Once you've identified which hand is stronger, hold the weaker hand still behind your partner's head and let the stronger hand move over the front of her head very slowly in a circular fashion (see fig. 3). *It is very important to move your hand clockwise from the point of view of an outside observer (even when treating yourself) because energy flows clockwise in the energy centers of the body. Again, do this slowly. A circle with a diameter of four inches should take four or five seconds to complete.*

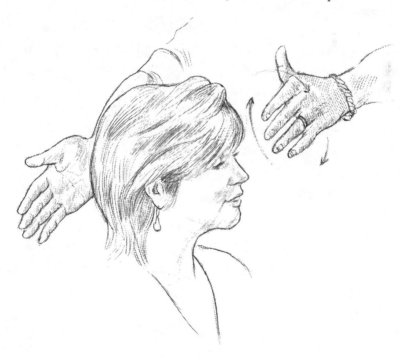

FIGURE 3

Start a half inch from your partner's head and very gradually move farther out. You'll feel different sensations in your hand as you move it, and different sensations say something about what is going on in the energy fields surrounding your partner's head and what to do about it. Tingling indicates an area of congested energy that requires a dose of your healing energy. A significant amount of congested energy of the type associated with extreme pain might make your hand buzz, perhaps even giving you a feeling of pins and needles in your hand and up your arm. This is natural and instructive, as it indicates where pain is concentrated. These sensations are a sign that you should deliver healing energy to this area until the sensations (tingling, buzzing, pins and needles, and so on) dissipate. If the buzzing goes all the way up to your elbow, however, pull away. This is too much negative energy for you to deal with at this point in your training.

As you work through the process of delivering energy to your partner's head, you will feel the buzzing ease and then get the sensation that the congestion is breaking up and releasing. As you do so, you will be lessening your partner's pain.

Another sensation to look for as you work is *no sensation at all*. A total absence of energy in the space around your partner's head would signal a significant depletion in energy in that area. This also warrants a strong dose of healing energy from you.

Remarkably, as soon as you learn to feel and develop the energy bubble, you can do a meaningful amount of healing work right away. Think of what a treat this will be for your spouse, child, best friend, or even your next-door neighbor the next time she mentions she has a stiff neck. You'll be the most popular person on your block in no time!

EXERCISE 3: FEELING THE BODY'S ENERGIES

Once you've created the energy bubble and used it to perform a basic level of healing on you or someone else, the next step is to learn to feel energies in different parts of the body. If you have a partner you can work with, start with this person.

Begin by calming your mind so you will be more aware of subtle shifts in your perception. I find that there are three methods for calming the mind that work for everyone.

- You can sit or stand very still, close your eyes, and concentrate on your breath as it flows in and out of your body for several moments.
- You can close your eyes and do a silent countdown from ten to one.
- You can imagine you are in a beautiful, tranquil place, perhaps somewhere you've been that makes you very peaceful.

Once you calm your mind, position your hands in a similar way you used them to heal in figure 3 and come in gently from the side, parallel to your partner's body. For the sake of this example, let's start with the shoulder (see fig. 4). Position your more powerful healing hand about one inch from the shoulder and slowly move it in a circular clockwise motion.

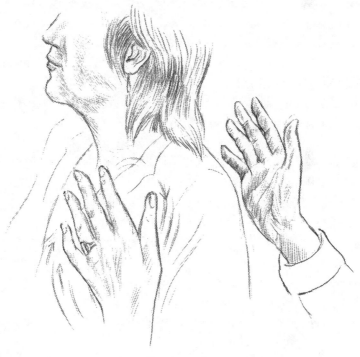

FIGURE 4

Notice what you feel. You might feel warmth, coolness, or something between. You should get some sense here that there is a subtle density of energy. It isn't important that you be able to read the messages of the energy at this point. Right now, the goal is to learn to identify it.

Now move your hand to the sternum area, heart-high. Slowly roll your hand clockwise here. Do you notice something different? You should get a sense that there is a great deal more energy here than there was near the shoulder (this is because you're close to one of the body's energy centers, which we'll discuss at length later).

Take ten minutes to scan your partner's body and feel the energies. You'll notice that these energies are different in different places—sometimes dramatically so. It's very possible that you'll feel pain in your hand when you do this. If the person you are scanning is carrying a high degree of pain somewhere in her body, this will come through to you. You will probably not be able to detect lower levels of pain at this point, though.

It might be a good idea at this stage to write down what you feel as you scan the energies in front of different body parts. Try to be as specific as possible, as this will provide a useful reference later.

EXERCISE 4: FEELING ENERGY INTERNALLY

Once you have some sense of how these energies feel in an external way, the next step is to learn to feel them internally. Later, you will learn how to use your body as a "photographic plate" to record someone else's energies. First, though, we're going to concentrate on the energies inside of you.

Lie down in your bed and make yourself as relaxed as possible. Use the same simple calming techniques we used for exercise 3 (focusing on your breathing, doing a ten-to-one silent countdown, or imagining that you are in a beautiful, peaceful place). The tool we're going to use here requires very careful focus of mental attention and awareness. Unlike feeling energy with your hands, you need to "send" your mind to different places in your body to feel these energies at an internal level. This requires you to focus your mental concentration on each of your various body parts, essentially putting a mental "searchlight" in each part.

We're moving up the ladder a bit with this exercise in terms of degree of difficulty. It is possible that you will not be able to do this immediately. Keep moving forward anyway. Remember that the goal of these early chapters is skill building. Stay with this process, keep working at it, and you'll feel your skills grow noticeably in a short period. Thousands of my clients have learned to do this with a little practice.

First, focus your attention on your right foot. What do you feel there? Do you get a sense of tingling or maybe a sense of warmth? The sensation should feel similar to the sensation you get in your hands when you use them to move energy. In this case, though, you will feel it from the inside.

Next, direct your attention to your right knee. You should feel less energy moving through your knee than your foot, unless you are under stress, in which case you will feel a high level of energy there. When stressed, we hold our bodies tight, and the stress in our muscles is telegraphed to the joints through tendons and ligaments. Knees are a place where we often carry this type of musculoskeletal tension.

From there, move to your right thigh. There's considerably less energy here, isn't there? That's because the thigh is not located near a major energy center in the body, so energy does not naturally collect here. However, you might feel strong energy moving through your thigh if you just exercised it or if it is injured. When you've taken note of this energy, move to your right hip. In what ways does this feel different?

Now feel the energies inside your entire body by taking the path illustrated in figure 5. Focusing your awareness on different body parts by following this path is easy. It amounts to scanning your bodily energies from the crown of your head, to the tip of your spine, down your extremities on the right, and then down the left side of the body. After you practice this path once or twice, it becomes second nature. As you practice, spend some time at each stop. Allow yourself to concentrate on and take note of what you are feeling. There are no rules in terms of the language you use to describe these feelings. Simply use whatever feels most comfortable and familiar to you and try to be consistent. Some people will describe the sensations in technical, logical terms. Others will use metaphors to describe the same feelings. The only important aspect is to develop your own consistent terminology. You want to be able to note similarities and differences between different parts of the body. You want to have a good understanding of your energy "baseline"—the energy pattern you are starting with—and you'll want to be able to describe changes that you feel from one day to the next as you begin to practice your healing skills.

Keep a record of your observations. Simplicity will do. Photocopy or trace the diagram of the human body from figure 5, or sketch your own

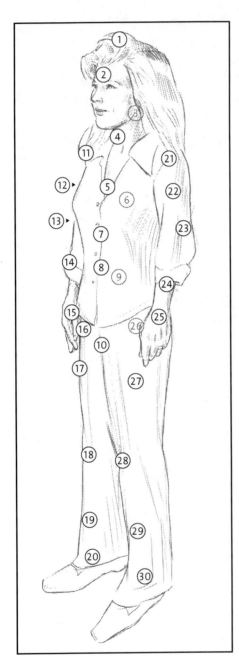

1. TOP OF HEAD
2. CENTER OF FOREHEAD
3. BACK OF THE HEAD WHERE IT MEETS THE SPINE
4. THROAT AND NECK
5. CENTER OF CHEST AT THE HEIGHT OF YOUR HEART
6. UPPER BACK
7. SOLAR PLEXUS
8. STOMACH
9. LOWER BACK
10. GENITALS
11. RIGHT SHOULDER
12. RIGHT UPPER ARM
13. RIGHT ELBOW
14. RIGHT FOREARM
15. RIGHT WRIST AND HAND
16. RIGHT HIP
17. RIGHT THIGH
18. RIGHT KNEE
19. RIGHT CALF
20. RIGHT ANKLE AND FOOT
21. LEFT SHOULDER
22. LEFT UPPER ARM
23. LEFT ELBOW
24. LEFT FOREARM
25. LEFT WRIST AND HAND
26. LEFT HIP
27. LEFT THIGH
28. LEFT KNEE
29. LEFT CALF
30. LEFT ANKLE AND FOOT

FIGURE 5

version, and write down a word or two of observation for each body site. Remake this map as you succeed in improving your diagnostic abilities and become more and more skilled as your own "biofield therapist." You're beginning an extraordinary journey of discovery here by learning the inner workings of your body, and you will soon learn how to have a genuine, positive impact on those workings.

EXERCISE 5: USING YOUR BODY TO FEEL ENERGY IN OTHERS (OPTIONAL)

When you've developed a strong familiarity with the energies in your own body, you're ready to learn how to use your body as a "photographic plate" to sense the energies in someone else's body. Obviously, this exercise is not necessary for your own health and healing, but you may find it highly rewarding and insightful to experiment with this method (and again, it'll make you a hit with your friends).

You'll need a partner for this. First, use one of the simple exercises we used earlier to calm and focus your mind. Then, stand in front of your partner, about four feet away. Stay in the same position for three or four minutes without moving to allow your partner's energy to seep into you. Notice what you feel throughout your body, performing the same kind of scan you performed on yourself when you were alone during exercise 4. Write your observations down and compare your notes to the notes from your latest personal scan. The differences you feel relate to the differences between your body's energy and the energy in your partner.

As was the case when you used your hands, you might feel a sense of pain if your partner has a high level of pain somewhere. Regardless, though, you should feel some differences over what you felt when you traced the energies of your own body. Again, it isn't important at this point that you understand what these differences mean. At this stage of skill building, it is only important that you learn to identify the differences and describe them to yourself in a consistent fashion.

YOUR TEN-DAY PLAN FOR DEVELOPING THESE SKILLS

These exercises are easy to perform and you will get an immediate "charge" out of each of them. Real skill comes with practice, however. If you work with these exercises every day for ten days, you will gain the level of skill necessary to move to the next level. If you found the first run-through exciting, imagine what it's going to be like in a couple of weeks. If you didn't get as much out of this as you hoped the first time around, keep going and you will tune in to your energies in dramatic ways.

The potency of these skills grows over time if you work at them a little each day because there will soon come a day when you will have astounding accuracy in your assessments and dramatic power to move energy for healing.

Work through this in stages. During the first five days, concentrate on the first three exercises (creating the energy bubble, using the bubble to move energy to another part of your body or a partner's body, and using your hands to feel the energy in a partner). After five days, continue to do the first three exercises daily and add the fourth exercise (the internal tour of your body's energies). You can experiment with the fifth exercise (using your body to feel the energy in others) at your leisure.

Have fun with this along the way. Practice your increasing ability to analyze another person's energy patterns by testing your skills with close friends, colleagues, or family members. Tell them you're learning the latest techniques in mind-body medicine and want to use them as "guinea pigs." Sense their energy patterns and venture to ask, for example, "Is your left knee bothering you?" Failure is as informative as success in the early stages of practicing these skills, so don't be shy. Practice on strangers without their even knowing it. When I first started, I practiced wherever I went. I would be in a mall, and as I passed shoppers, I would scan them energetically (keeping my observations to myself, of course).

The practice is what's important. The mind, to some degree, is a kinesthetic instrument; it learns by doing. Practice these skills wherever you can, as much as you can.

Always keep your goals in mind, too. You are teaching yourself to have an impact on your health and wellbeing that you've never had before. As each chapter of this book passes, you are getting closer to making your own mind the most skillful and compassionate "doctor" you've ever met.

PRELUDE TO 3

A HYPNOTIC HOLIDAY

L et's begin with a quick exercise that will demonstrate the extraordinary power of hypnosis—a second tool to add to your energy skills. Before you begin this exercise, however, pay close attention to how your body feels right now. Sense whether you're in pain, stressed, or drained and whether you're worried about it. Are you feeling anxious or maybe "you're not all there?" Now rate the overall level of distress in your body and mind. Use the same one-to-ten scale you used earlier: a one is "I'm feeling fine," and a ten is "Could someone please shoot me and put me out of my misery?"

Next, prepare for this exercise in the same way you prepared for the exercises at the starts of chapters 1 and 2. Turn off the phone, sit back comfortably, close your eyes, and begin to monitor your breath going in and out. Feel yourself calm. Then, begin counting slowly backwards from ten to one. When you reach one, you're ready to begin.

Now imagine the following:

You are going to the airport to get on a plane and fly off for a well-deserved vacation. The airport is amazingly easy to get through—no lines and no problem with security—and the flight isn't crowded. Maybe they even offer you a glass of wine or dessert, courtesy of the airline. Everything is going great. Your fantastic vacation is just the way you planned it: the perfect Caribbean holiday. You've been looking forward to this day for ages—away from the world, away from the distractions.

Now imagine checking into your five-star resort hotel. You love your room. You are now walking out to the beach. You smell the food from the restaurant. You have your bathing suit on and you have your towel. You pick out a lounge chair by the sea. There is sun, but not too much. You can feel the sand under your feet. "Aaahhh," you know the feeling. You look out over the water, and it's magnificent—a cerulean blue with the sunlight dancing on it. The sky is clear with a few white puffy clouds skipping along the horizon. Children are going happily by. Birds are singing and soaring about. It is heaven on earth. You lie back on your lounge chair and say, "I deserve it." You draw in a deep breath and relax. It feels so great.

You want to go in the water, so you get up lazily and wade into the water, and it's delightful. Maybe you splash and swim around a little. This is the kind of day where there is nothing to do but have a good time, and so you do. You take a little nap, and afterward, you think of the restaurant. It smells pretty darn good, and you stroll into the restaurant to have a magnificent meal. After that, you say, "What the heck; I'm going to have a massage." The resort has a spa, and you get a professional massage on a private terrace overlooking the water. Your body hasn't felt this good in a long, long time.

After that, you wander back out on the beach for a stroll. You realize this vacation is even more lavish and refreshing than you thought it would be. This is one of the best vacations in your life. You say to yourself, "Boy, booking this vacation is the smartest thing I've done in years."

Now, open your eyes and notice how your body and mind feel. Rate yourself again on that one-to-ten scale. You'll probably find you feel much, much better than before. That's because you just entered a light hypnotic state and cut your stress dramatically. This is just a tiny example of what hypnosis can do for you, both physically and mentally.

Let's take that up to an entirely different level right now.

CHAPTER 3

HYPNOSIS

About five years ago, a busy middle-aged African-American female physician came to see me, stressed and utterly disorganized. She'd gotten to the point where she was even having trouble keeping pace with her career. We spoke for a while and slowly came around to the part of her story that was causing her problem. She was the first generation in her family to go to college and attain an upper-class lifestyle. Carrying the family mantle in a world where she had to be so much better than her white peers just to make the grade gradually took its toll on her. At our second appointment, she arrived with a terrible migraine headache and confessed she'd been plagued with chronic migraines for years. How she drove to my office, I'll never know. During that second session, I took her into hypnosis, conducted a progressive relaxation exercise to relieve her stress (you'll learn this later in the book), then threw in some imagery designed to free her from the migraine. When the session ended, she opened her eyes and said, "My migraine's gone."

The migraines never returned.

A PRIMER ON HYPNOSIS

Unless you've been involved with hypnosis before, there's an excellent chance what you think you know about it is wrong. Let me dispel a few notions immediately:

- Hypnosis will not leave you quacking like a duck during an important meeting. There's a huge difference between stage hypnotism (an entertainment medium) and therapeutic hypnosis, which is what we're going to be doing.
- Hypnosis will not put you under the control of another person. You will be in control the entire time.
- Hypnosis does not involve the loss of awareness. In fact, the opposite is true—your awareness is very sharp and you always know what is happening.
- Hypnosis does not involve a loss of memory. You'll remember everything that happens while you are hypnotized.
- It isn't true that some people can't be hypnotized. Everyone can be hypnotized and benefit from the power of hypnosis.

Therapeutic hypnosis is simply a tool that lets you focus your awareness on thoughts, feelings, insights, and sensory experiences normally hidden from view. Psychologists use the metaphor of the searchlight to describe the focus of the mind's awareness (as I did in the last chapter). The skill of hypnosis will allow you to focus the searchlight of your awareness so you can understand yourself better and uncover some of the hidden messages that have been driving your life—and having a strong influence on your health and wellbeing.

Before I can teach you how to use hypnosis effectively, though, I need to talk to you a little about what your mind is capable of doing.

THE HIDDEN POWER OF THE MIND

Human awareness has three levels: the conscious mind, the subconscious mind, and the super-conscious mind. Each of these levels of awareness has different content, and you access each using a different type of thinking.

Your conscious mind consists of your everyday perceptions, thoughts, attitudes, and feelings—the facets about yourself of which you are very much aware. Your conscious mind "speaks" to you in your native language as analytical thought or reason. You are well aware of your conscious mind already, as this part of your mind is with you through all of your waking hours.

The subconscious mind is a hidden storehouse of memories, deep feelings, desires and aspirations, motives, knowledge, and other intensely meaningful aspects of you of which you are *not* usually aware. The subconscious mind is gigantic in size and power compared to the conscious mind. Sigmund Freud's model of human consciousness looked like an iceberg, with conscious mind at the tip (the part you can see above the water) and subconscious mind enormous but hidden (the part submerged under water).

The subconscious mind has numerous functions. It plays a role in guiding your bodily processes: your heartbeat, circulation, immune functioning, and so forth. It also contains a library-like catalogue of your life experiences and the thoughts and feelings associated with your important events. You probably can't recall what you were doing, feeling, and thinking on New Year's Eve when you were five years old, but your subconscious mind has it all tucked away in living color with surround sound.

Even with all of this, there is still more to the subconscious mind. Carl Jung, Freud's colleague, first coined the phrase "the collective unconscious" to describe an aspect of subconscious awareness that includes a storehouse of latent memory traces from man's ancestral past—the whole history of our evolution. We can tap into this universal component of human consciousness through the subconscious mind. Included in the collective unconscious are "archetypes," basic human personality patterns that we live out. These are personality roles—warrior, caregiver, seeker, sage, fool, and so on. How many people do you know who live life like a battle that needs to be won, or are always going around taking care of everyone else, or always on an adventure? These people are subconsciously filling various archetypal roles. In hypnotic work, we access these archetypal patterns to promote healing, often with miraculous results.

The subconscious mind is *extremely aware*, even when the conscious mind is asleep at the wheel. Have you ever pulled into the driveway and wondered just how you got there because you don't remember the drive home? Your conscious mind was so focused on something—a report that's due, for example—that you made the entire trip thinking about only that. Who drove the car? Your subconscious mind. In fact, your subconscious mind does anything you do by rote memory—standing, walking, taking a shower, and so forth.

The subconscious mind "communicates" using symbolic thoughts—deep feelings, stories, myths, and metaphors. The most powerful tool you can employ to tap its power is hypnosis. Hypnosis literally opens a vast new world to you.

Getting in touch with your subconscious mind will help you accomplish two things. First, you can discover and release old trauma, emotional pain, or distorted beliefs that might be keeping illness in your body (remember the stories of Erin's miscarriages and John's near-blindness). Second, you can access your archetypal understanding of who you are and what your true role in life is.

A good third of my patients encountered poor health because they were leading lives that were inauthentic to their deepest self-aspirations. They weren't doing this deliberately, but they were doing it because they weren't effectively in touch with their subconscious minds.

For example, in 1994, a woman in her early thirties from Washington, D.C., came to see me for help with advanced degenerative disc disease. She was living with excruciating levels of pain that no prescription painkiller could touch. After two surgeries and months of physical therapy, her doctors had done all they could for her. Since she was still in tremendous amounts of pain, this was not nearly enough. I used biofield therapy to alleviate her pain, but to find a cure for her problem, we had to get to the underlying cause of the disease. Under hypnosis, this young woman's subconscious played out the archetypal "story" that she was a priestly healer (she was currently a senior-level bureaucrat for the United States Public Health Service, the last in a long line of generations of her family who had been public servants). On the strength of the self-knowledge she gained under hypnosis, she went back to graduate school, got a degree in theology, and became a priest. At the same time, the disease arrested. As a result, she became truly happy because she started living a life that was authentic to her most deeply held desires—desires she didn't really understand until she discovered them under hypnosis.

The third level of human awareness is the super-conscious mind, which is literally infinite in power. I mean this—it has no limits. Once you access super-conscious awareness and learn to "steer" it, you can heal yourself and others and accomplish just about anything you want in life. The super-conscious mind exists at two levels: the individual super-conscious mind and the universal super-conscious mind.

The individual super-conscious mind is a level of "thought" or consciousness capable of sensing and influencing electromagnetic energy fields. Using this level of thought, we have the power to direct our own personal electromagnetic energy fields (the BioEM energies discussed in chapter 2), as well as the electromagnetic energy fields around us. By the way of the individual super-conscious mind, you can improve your health, your environment, and your future to a much greater degree than you might believe right now. The form of thought that is required to access the individual super-conscious mind is intuitive thought—a deep, immediate, and accurate sense of knowing something that we could not necessarily know through simple logic.

A vast majority of people have had an intuitive experience. If you're a parent, perhaps you've awakened in the middle of the night with a nagging fear that something is wrong with your daughter who is away at college. You call her the next day to find out that she's sick or upset. If you've been through something like this, you've experienced intuitive thought.

Two summers ago, I was traveling in the state of Washington on vacation, flying up the coast highway through one majestic stand of timber after another. Suddenly, for no obvious reason, I began to feel very ill at ease. I came up over the next rise, saw hundreds of acres of forest on both sides of the highway that had been clear-cut by the logging industry, and immediately understood what my intuition was trying to tell me.

Intuitive thought is a subtle form of awareness most people don't "hear" because of all the loud static carried in our minds and the surrounding environment. It is nonetheless present in all people, and you can develop it to a high degree of sophistication. I will introduce you to the skills you'll require to experience it before the close of this chapter.

The intuitive thought of the individual super-conscious mind is a gateway to an even larger field of intelligent energy that I call the universal super-conscious mind. To understand it, let's look at it first through the lens of science, then through the inspiration of faith—two different means of comprehending the same extraordinary reality.

For the scientific perspective, we turn to the work of the great physicists: Albert Einstein, Neils Bohr, and John Stuart Bell, who proved that there is a single, mammoth conscious energy field that exists back behind the near infinite number of individual electromagnetic energy fields that make up the entire universe. Scientists call this reality the unified field, a single field that behaves in predictable, elegant, intelligent ways to create and sustain the entire universe. Within this field, each thing in the universe is instantaneously connected to and reacting with everything else. From this perspective, you can see the unified field as one vast universal "thought" that directs the form and function of everything in existence.

This is the only explanation for the precision and perfection evident in the way things operate. Brian Green, a Nobel laureate in physics, compares the universe to an epic novel and the unified field to the creativity and strategy of its author, saying that any attempt to understand the universe armed only with the tools of science as we know it is like trying to understand a Tolstoy novel armed only with the rules of grammar.

When I describe the "scientific perspective" to an audience, invariably someone of deep faith raises a hand and says, "Oh yes, there is a thought behind the universe all right. It's God's thought." Religious thinkers of many faiths have long maintained that the universe exists as a thought held in the mind of God. As a man of science and faith, and as someone who spends a great deal of time in super-conscious levels of awareness, I couldn't agree more.

Both perspectives—that of science and of faith—have great merit. Both have something to offer regarding the search for ultimate meaning, and each needs the point of view of the other. Religious people have a lot going for them. They tend to have an unlimited view of what goes on "outside the box," rightly assert there is a larger purpose playing out there, and are hungry to find it. However, they too often pay more attention to chapter and verse than to direct experience. That's where science comes in. Science is new to exploring the hidden power of the mind but is very good at establishing "fact" as it arises out of direct experience. The inspiration provided by faith, coupled with the objective realism of science, provides an efficient means for exploring the greatest remaining frontier of human understanding—the mind.

Whether you are a scientific humanist or a person of deep faith, you can reach universal super-conscious awareness via meditative thought. Meditative thought opens up the part of your awareness that lets you experience yourself as "one" with the universal super-conscious mind. Think of the universal super-consciousness mind as a vast ocean and your individual super-consciousness as a wave on this ocean. The wave is of the same substance as the ocean and always connected to it, even when it makes a big splash on the beach. I will teach you how to reach meditative thought later. For now, the important thing to realize is that an aspect of your mind exists in constant communion with the entire universe. When you learn to experience this power, you will enjoy levels of health, peace, and joy exponentially greater than what most people imagine.

In 1995, a professional colleague of mine called me to ask for an emergency appointment. She'd just come from her surgeon's office where she learned she had a "highly suspicious" mass in her left breast that a mammogram and ultrasound indicated could be cancerous. The mass was so dense that her surgeon broke two biopsy needles during his examination. She had a history of breast cancer in her family, so the odds were against her. Her surgeon had her scheduled for a lumpectomy two days hence, and they both agreed he would perform a mastectomy if the mass was cancerous, which seemed very likely.

I met her at my office at 5:00 the next morning. I used hypnosis to guide her into super-conscious awareness—a hypnotically induced state of deep meditation—where she remained for about forty-five minutes. When she opened her eyes, she was smiling.

"What was that?" she asked. "I've never experienced such peace and joy. I was in my body and outside of it at the same time. From outside my body, I watched the tumor in my breast just dissolve away."

Two days later when she woke up in post-op, her surgeon was sitting bedside. Shaking his head, he said, "I don't understand it. I've never seen anything like it in all my years of surgery. There was nothing there. Go back to sleep dear, you do not have cancer."

THE REVELATORY POWER OF HYPNOSIS

By learning and developing your skills at hypnosis, you can focus the searchlight of your awareness in very powerful ways to uncover the content of your subconscious and super-conscious minds.

Typically, a psychological wall stops what is in the subconscious mind from going into the conscious mind, and vice versa. In psychology, this wall is known as a "gatekeeper." Hypnosis moves the gatekeeper out of the way by calming the mind, at which point the gatekeeper simply relaxes and slides out of the way, allowing you to have access to the content of your conscious and subconscious minds at the same time. There's a second gatekeeper between the subconscious and super-conscious minds. Deep hypnotic states and advanced states of meditation drop this gatekeeper out of the way, at which point you can naturally perceive the intuitive thought that opens you to super-conscious awareness. (We'll get to this later.)

Because hypnosis allows you to uncover what you have hidden in the subconscious and super-conscious minds, it gives you perfect insight into your *story behind the story*, an essential discovery on the path to healing. It will dramatically reduce stress in the mind and body and give you more power for healing than you've ever had before.

One of the huge advantages of hypnosis is its value as a stress-reduction tool. Physical and psychological stress causes 50 percent of all disease and mortality. If you are already suffering from ill health—especially if you suffer from conditions like heart disease, cancer, diabetes, asthma, arthritis, fibromyalgia, hypertension, ulcers, and certain neurological disorders—you cannot afford stress. Hypnosis will provide you with a solution.

In addition, stress is often a major contributor to chronic illness. If you know someone with a genetic predisposition to diseases like heart disease or diabetes who has managed to sidestep this proclivity, it's likely he or she does a good job managing stress. The same is true with injuries. Research indicates that injuries tend to locate in particular areas of the body where a person holds stress. One tennis player will tear a rotator cuff while another stays healthy largely because the first player stored too much stress in the shoulder, making it susceptible to injury.

Because of its power, hypnosis lies at the heart of many of the healing plans in this book. It is so undeniably powerful that you can use it in a seemingly endless number of ways to improve your physical and mental health. First, though, you need to get good enough at it to utilize it effectively.

WHAT TO EXPECT

People will naturally go into hypnosis and enjoy its benefits when they know what to expect. Some people wonder, "What if I can't be hypnotized?" or "What if I screw it up?" Relax. Everyone can be hypnotized and you can't screw it up. Hypnosis is a naturally occurring state of awareness. While you may not know it, you are often in a hypnotic state. You're in a light state of hypnosis when focused on a task to such an extent that you are unaware of what's going on around you. People who sit in a busy airport terminal pounding away on their laptops while oblivious to the noise are in light hypnosis. If you've ever had the experience of spacing out while driving, maybe intending to go to a friend's house and winding up at the grocery store instead, you've experienced medium hypnosis. Everyone enters a state of deep hypnosis just before falling asleep and just before waking up. We all go into hypnosis naturally and often. What I'll help you do is control how and when you go into hypnosis and teach you how to use it to achieve your goals for health and wellbeing.

Later in this book, I will present you with the hypnotic pre-talk I provide all of my patients. This will give you extensive detail on what to expect. For the sake of the skill building exercises in this chapter however, you just need to know the basics:

- Your attention will shift more directly into yourself and away from your environment. This is a function of focusing, as would be the case with concentrating on a challenging task.
- Though you will be more aware of what you experience in yourself than the surrounding environment, you will still be aware of the outside world. You'll still hear loud noises or feel the presence of others who might come into the room.
- The process will make you feel very relaxed. You will go deeper—and make the most of the experience—if you adopt a highly receptive attitude. Follow the process, and you'll get a big payoff.
- Once in a hypnotic state, you will experience thoughts, feelings, and images moving through your mind. However, people differ in how these impressions arise. For some, most of what the mind presents will be in the form of thought. For some, it is imagery, which can be very vague,

or sharp and powerful, somewhat like watching a movie. Many people see, feel, and hear things. Some even experience smell and taste.

GOING IN

Hypnosis requires something known as an induction, a formalized group of words, phrases, and imagery that moves your attention away from the outside world and toward a relaxed and focused inner awareness. This process naturally moves you past the gatekeeper.

I will provide the inductions you use here and elsewhere in the book. These inductions are available at www.miraculoushealthbook.com as downloads. I'm providing these inductions for you for two reasons. The first is that, when you perform the induction yourself, you're trying to do two things at once, which is going to distract you. You need to become considerably more familiar with this process before you can do the inductions effectively. The second reason is that I am a board-certified hypnotherapist. I know how to use voice inflection and move energies through my voice to carry you deeper into hypnosis than you would go if you made a recording of your own voice from a scripted induction.

There are many inductions available for download from my website, and these are free to purchasers of this book. Certain types of inductions work better for particular personality types. Inductions also vary depending on the type of work you intend to do while under hypnosis. As I walk you through the following chapters, I will guide you in selecting the inductions that are best for you. I will also encourage you to experiment with different induction techniques until you find the process that works best. However, for the purposes of this chapter, we'll stick with the basics. You'll be utilizing my most popular induction methods for now and will get a lot out of these if you know what to expect.

The inductions I often use have three parts. The first part is a basic focusing and relaxing procedure, often a ten-to-one countdown using a variety of voice modulations and prompts. The second part is a bodily relaxation procedure. I typically use progressive relaxation, which involves imagining a warm, relaxing, and comfortable feeling starting in the tips of the toes and going all the way to the top of the head. Sometimes I use a "Jacobsonian" approach, directing you to tense and then release tension in various parts of your body. This approach works better for people who carry a lot of stress.

The third part of the induction uses imagery to draw you deeper in and prepare your mind for the particular work you are going to do (which I discuss at length in subsequent chapters). Imagery focuses your attention further while at the same time stimulating your senses. I might take you to the beach and have you feel the texture of the sand, see the color of the sky, hear the sounds of the water, and smell the salt in the air. This type of induction serves to heighten bodily awareness, and I might choose to use it if the purpose of your hypnotic session was to release physical pain. Alternatively, I might suggest during the induction that you imagine your body filling with white light and then melting into that light. I would choose a white light induction if the purpose of your work for this session is to take you into super-conscious states of awareness. Over the course of this book, you'll have the opportunity to work with a variety of my induction styles. As you gain more practice with hypnosis, you'll find which of these feel best to you and offer you the most rewarding experience.

It's time to start your journey.

EXERCISE 1: EXPERIENCING HYPNOSIS

The first skill to learn is entering and exiting a hypnotic state. Download Induction Alpha-I from www.miraculoushealthbook.com. Burn this download onto a CD so you can play it in a room where it will be easy for you to relax.

Before you begin any hypnosis session, always check your bladder. You do not want to have to get up in the middle of this, as you'll lose much of the power of the experience if you do. More importantly, make sure to leave yourself enough time at the end of the session to walk around for a few minutes before driving or operating any kind of machinery. Hypnosis calms the body, slows the heart rate, and draws the mind into deep, peaceful awareness. When you come out of it, you will enjoy a relaxed languid feeling, much as you would after a nice massage. You might feel a little spacey, and your reflexes will be a little slower. You'll want to enjoy this as much as possible, so avoid beginning a session if you need to run out of the house immediately afterward. Also, be sure not to drink alcohol or coffee immediately before your session.

Now turn off the phone and situate yourself in a room free of disturbances and interruptions. Dim the lights and turn off background music, such as television or anything of this sort. Lie down in a bed or stretch out on a sofa or in a comfortable chair (see fig. 6). Recline enough to relax completely and not have to exert any effort to hold your head up. Many people like to have a blanket over them as well.

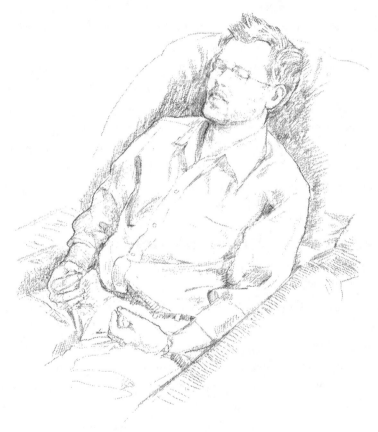

FIGURE 6

Turn on the CD and listen as I guide you through the process. We'll move through the three stages of induction I've already described and then, after a few minutes, into a brief "emerging" technique that will guide you back to normal waking awareness. The entire session will last approximately fifteen minutes and will leave you feeling peaceful and refreshed.

One of the wonderful things about the "work" you'll be doing with hypnosis—and later with meditation—is that it is a deeply pleasurable experience. You'll gain important skills if you put in the effort, but you will feel the benefits right away. If you've ever had the experience of needing to practice something you really love—tennis, cooking, or guitar, for instance—you'll know what I'm talking about.

It is possible you will not be able to immediately relax mentally. If this happens, it is likely you feel some sense of resistance to the process. You may not be aware of this on a conscious level, but something is preventing you from getting past the gatekeeper. People who are tightly controlled might have to practice the process a few times before they are able to relax mentally. If this happens to you, it's okay. You'll learn something valuable that you will use when we get into self-analysis and treatment. All it means is that you are going through a different hypnotic experience—the opportunity to uncover your defense mechanisms and the source of your stress. You'll learn ways to get around this later in the book.

Another experience you might encounter when you start to relax is that you might fall asleep. This is an indication that your resources are depleted, maybe dramatically so. If you fall asleep, you won't get the benefit of hypnosis, but you will get the benefit of something else—much needed rest. Take advantage of it. Then come back the next day and the one after that, as many days as necessary to begin your hypnosis training. Be aware that some people think they are asleep when they are not. The experience of hypnosis can mimic sleep because the mind and body go into a perfect restful state of peace. If you come back at the end of the exercise, aware of my voice prompting you to awaken and open your eyes, then you were not asleep. If, however, you come around half an hour after the exercise has ended (long after my voice prompts have ended), then you were asleep.

If you have a physical injury or a debilitating disease, the pain from this might make it harder to relax. Do not worry if you find you cannot relax physically or feel distracted because of pain in your body. Just keep trying. Mental relaxation is not the same as physical relaxation. With a little practice, you'll learn to focus on the induction and relax your mind. The upside is that you will move your attention away from the pain in order to relax into the induction and also begin effecting advance treatment in the area where you feel pain. In later sections of the book, we'll use deep hypnosis to address pain and tension in the body.

Use the Alpha-I induction every day for five days (do not skip any days). As I said, this will be some of the most enjoyable "work" you've ever done.

You will then be ready to move to exercise 2.

EXERCISE 2: FEELING ENERGY WHILE IN A HYPNOTIC STATE

By now, you should have ten days or more of practice using the skills taught in chapter 2, where you learned to feel the BioEM energies in and around your body. When you go through this process while in a hypnotic state, you'll experience these energies more accurately and gain a much clearer picture of what is going on in your body. This is so because under hypnosis, the "searchlight" of your awareness is very keen, the mind much more sensitive—you'll be able to perceive subtle sensations under hypnosis that you didn't notice in a conscious waking state.

Download Induction Alpha-II from www.miraculoushealthbook.com. As before, burn this download onto a CD so you can play it in a room where it will be easy to relax. This second induction is somewhat different from the first because the goal now is to focus on feeling energies in the body. We will move through the body in a similar way to exercise 4 in chapter 2 (beginning at the top of the head and moving through each part of the body until you've focused the searchlight of your attention on every body part). You will come away from this with a powerful new sense of how energies are moving through your body. As I take you through the process in the download, I will give you an idea of what to look for.

After each session, spend a few minutes writing about what you felt. Photocopy or sketch the silhouette of the human body from chapter 2 and make notes regarding your observations about the sensations in various body parts. This is important; otherwise, it will be difficult to remember later how the experience changed from session to session. Over time, you'll note a progression and see that your sense of the energies in your body, both under hypnosis and while in a normal conscious state, is considerably more acute than when you began.

This is a tremendously valuable bit of skill building. It isn't important to interpret what you've written at this point. That will come when we get to diagnosis and treatment. What is important is that you hone your sensitivity to your bodily energies and their related sensations. Doing so will serve you very well.

YOUR TEN-DAY PLAN FOR DEVELOPING SKILL IN HYPNOSIS

As with the energy exercises in chapter 2, you will develop real skill at using the tool of hypnosis through practice. Work through this in two simple stages. Practice the first exercise (Induction Alpha-I) for five days. For the following five days, add the second exercise (Induction Alpha-II). If you practice the techniques every day, you will gain the level of skill necessary to move to the next chapter and continue your journey to health.

Some of you will become an expert almost overnight in the use of this tool while some of you will take a bit longer. Whatever your initial experience with the exercises in this chapter, their potency will grow with practice. You will "slide" quickly and deeply into hypnosis with repeated exposure to the process.

If you can, continue practicing the energy exercises from chapter 2 during this time, as well. These tools compliment one another. The power and benefit of any one tool is bolstered by practicing the others you have in your kit. You should also notice a positive health benefit right away—a reduction in pain, improved stamina, and lower blood pressure, for example—even though the most exciting and rewarding work of self-assessment and treatment is still ahead.

Prelude to 4

An Instant Stressbuster

This brief exercise will give you a glimpse into the remarkable benefit meditation can bring to your life. Before you start, pay close attention to how your body is feeling right now, the same way you did with the exercises that preceded chapters 1 and 3. Do you feel any pain or stress? Is some physical ailment nagging you? Once again, rate the overall level of distress in your body and mind. Use the same one-to-ten scale: a one is "I'm doing great," and a ten is "I didn't know it was possible for a person to feel this miserable."

Once again, relax and focus your mind. Turn off the phone, sit back, close your eyes, and allow yourself to get comfortable. Start to monitor your breath going in and out. Don't force the breath or time it in any way; just observe it go in and out on its own for a few breaths, concentrating exclusively on the flow of breath. Next, begin silently counting backwards from ten to one. Count slowly, waiting about three seconds between each number. Now you're ready to begin.

Focus again on your breath. Remember, you're not trying to control it. Just let it flow naturally. Now each time your breath goes out, silently say "out" for the length of the out-breath. If you drift off a little bit, no big deal, just come back to the process. Do this for about five minutes.

Stop and open your eyes. Notice how you feel. You should notice that you feel somewhat better in your mind and body because you've entered into a light meditative state and significantly cut your physical and mental stress. Whatever your physical concern is, you'll notice the condition has improved, and not just a little—most people find that this simple exercise makes them feel a good deal better. My guess is that after you've had this little taste, you're going to want this feeling in your life all the time. If you can feel this much better after just a few minutes, imagine what's possible when you do this regularly.

At this point, it does not matter whether the effect of this first exercise lasts or not. What matters is what you've just experienced—a tiny sample of the stress-reducing, health-affirming power of meditation. Over time, the right use of meditation can deliver permanent, often miraculous benefits to your physical and mental health. It will also give you a stronger sense of spiritual wellbeing than you've had before.

Meditation is a remarkable thing. Let's show you how to make it a valuable part of your life.

CHAPTER 4

MEDITATION

I grew up in Bethesda, Maryland, went to one of the top public high schools in the country, and graduated fifth in my class of about 750 students. As a teenager, I was hardworking and frankly, a little neurotic. Both of my parents were scientists. My father (an internationally prominent biochemist) trained me to view the world in a hard-nosed, empirical fashion. Science and public service were his mantra, and he brought me up to think the same way. My fond childhood memories are not of the smell of home-baked bread but of the acrid perfumes of a chemistry lab. Back then, if you asked me about my religious beliefs, I might have said I was an agnostic. In other words, I wasn't the most likely candidate in the world to embrace spirituality.

I went off to Brandeis University in 1966, determined to get an MD and PhD and follow in my father's footsteps. Brandeis was a crucible for radical thought at that time, and much to my parents' chagrin, I became somewhat of a radical proponent for social change. The larger world was in trouble, and I didn't believe I could help solve the problems by making another breakthrough in biochemistry. So I traded in my white shirt and tie for fatigues and long hair and spearheaded a number of anti-discrimination and anti-war efforts.

Then, in 1969, Dr. Richard Alpert, now known as Baba Ram Dass, returned to the United States from a long trip to India to become one of the major teachers of Eastern thought and meditation in this country. His father was one of the founders of Brandeis and when Ram Dass returned, he gave two lectures in a class I was taking in the Sociology Department.

Ram Dass was quite the sight in his robe and sandals with a big beard and long hair. Even in the late sixties, this was unusual. When he started talking, he became more of an anomaly. He spoke of the infinite power of the human mind and of his experiences in India, where his guru regularly demonstrated the ability to foresee the future, heal the sick, change events, and otherwise defy the limits of time and space. He taught a simple meditative technique as a means to access this power and claimed it existed in every human being. His personal charisma was overwhelming.

That first seminar with Ram Dass touched me deeply. It was as if it awoke a sleeping giant within me. I'd never experienced anything like the joy that bubbled up in my heart and mind when I heard him speak. Ram Dass stirred my soul and changed my direction. I knew at that point meditation would become a regular part of my life. The rigorous scientist/social reformer had discovered the liberating qualities of spirit.

I was fortunate to meet Ram Dass when I did. Not long after he came to Brandeis, he became a nationally known spiritual leader with thousands camped out daily on his father's estate to hear him speak. However, before his fame made him inaccessible, three or four of my classmates and I would spend half a day with him, listening to him talk and meditating together. Just by being in his presence, I felt my connection to something larger than myself. It was a palpable feeling of love and expansiveness I couldn't get enough of. After a few trips, we decided to start taking a skeptic along with us every time we went. The doubter-of-the-day would walk into the room and feel the energy in the place. Invariably, within five minutes that person would be crying tears of release and joy.

My early experiences with Ram Dass underscored a critical point: meditation is incredibly good for you and can make the seemingly impossible possible.

MEDITATION IS FOR *EVERYONE*

Meditation might well be the single most effective means you have available to effect your health and happiness. A couple of years ago, *Time* magazine did a major article on meditation, noting that it was "no longer for people with crystals." Meditation now has more than seventeen million practitioners in the United States, people of every age, culture, faith, and philosophy. Why? Because it delivers a wide range of benefits that make you feel better, more connected, and more alive than you ever thought possible.

Researchers in the health and allied-health sciences have identified a huge array of therapeutic benefits that derive from meditation. It improves rates of recovery from a variety of illnesses, especially those with a strong mental component, such as asthma, arthritis, fibromyalgia, heart disease, hypertension, and ulcers. Dr. Dean Ornish's combination of diet and meditation has had proven effect in reducing plaque in the arteries—diet alone doesn't do it, but the combination of meditation and diet does. Dr. Jon Kabat-Zinn has employed meditation effectively on cancer, immune problems, and many other types of chronic and debilitating health concerns, demonstrating conclusively that meditation improves circulation, vitality, stamina and resistance to disease. It is instrumental in the management of chronic pain. Indeed, it can wipe out chronic pain altogether.

Meditation has an enormously positive impact on physical health. I've seen it with my patients, and I've also seen it with myself. My grandfather on my father's side died of a massive heart attack when he was sixty-one. My father had a major heart attack when he was fifty-five. By my late forties, I began to develop serious heart problems: high blood pressure, an arrhythmia, and bouts of angina. This was my genetic fate, something that was predestined to happen to my body. I was fully aware of my genetic predisposition. I was equally aware that I was complicating the problem by carrying too much emotional pain in my heart.

Cardiac surgeons at Johns Hopkins have observed that their heart surgery patients tend to be people who have suffered massive losses of love in their lives. We tend to attach love issues to the heart because the heart symbolizes love in our culture. If we have lost in love, we might say, "My heart is broken." People suffering a break-up will often experience physical heart pain, and so on. Simply put, people who've experienced love loss tend to store the resulting painful emotional energy in the heart.

This described me perfectly. I was in a massive amount of emotional pain from a long-term marriage that I was completely committed to—my values as a person wouldn't let me walk away no matter the difficulties—and I'd been feeling this pain for many years. I took it on willingly as a means to carry my wife's burdens and to shield my children from the unrest that would have resulted had I refused to suffer in silence. So many people elect to make the same sacrifice for their loved ones. Perhaps the only thing distinguishing me from the average person was that I knew *exactly* what I was doing and what the consequences would be.

I carried this emotional pain in my heart until my children had gone to college. Then I set to work healing myself, knowing it might mean the end of my marriage. Some of the work involved dealing with the relationship. That part of the journey was complicated, involved years of effort, and not surprisingly, increased the negative emotional energy in and around my heart. I healed myself exclusively through meditation. I would go into deep meditation daily where I would focus on healing both my physical heart and my emotional pain. Sometimes this exploration would bring me to tears.

I continued to meditate in this way for about a year. I lowered my blood pressure, stopped feeling pain in my chest, and increased my endurance. At about that time, I went for a cardiac stress test and when it was over, my cardiologist said, "Wow, Rick, your heart is functioning at the level of a professional athlete. It looks like you avoided the family curse." I healed my physical heart through the power of meditation, even though the problems in my marriage persisted. You can heal yourself using meditation too, even if your circumstances remain difficult.

Meditation also has a number of mental and spiritual benefits, which invariably have an impact on physical health. It substantially reduces fear, anxiety, and depression, all of which precede or accompany chronic health problems.

Meditation is the perfect salve for stress. Stress causes 50 percent of what kills us and 50 percent of what chronically disables us. If you suffer from physical health problems, you simply can't afford stress. Fortunately, you've come to the right place for this because I have the ideal tool for you to use to reduce stress.

Meditation delivers greater mental clarity, peace of mind, and optimism. It will also bring you profound intuitive insights regarding your physical and mental health, as well as provide answers to questions regarding the meaning and purpose of life—insights critical to getting to your *story behind the story*. If you so choose, you can use meditation to move into expansive states of spiritual awareness, a worthy ideal for the person of faith and the scientific humanist alike.

Clearly, meditation is a gift from the gods for people with health problems. It is also so easy a child can do it.

So why isn't everyone meditating?

There are two reasons why more people don't meditate. The first has to do with our cultural conditioning. Everything in our society urges us to "go out there and conquer the world," and we're all very busy trying to make that happen. Taking the time to go inward in silence so you can heal yourself and achieve your goals seems counter-intuitive. However, it works. I've converted many hard-working rationalists to the ease and potency of meditation—among them, some of the busiest, most powerful people in the world (who subsequently have become less busy and more powerful). You too can have this experience if you open yourself up to it.

The second reason is that some people are under the impression meditation is difficult. Now, I grant you that a few dyed-in-the-wool Type A overachievers have difficulty relaxing enough to meditate when they first try it. However, everyone can meditate effectively—and easily—with the right methods and an understanding of what to expect.

It is absolutely worth doing a little work now to learn these methods. The benefits are huge. Meditation will free you from the box you're living in, grant you the power you need to heal yourself, and exponentially expand your ability to get what you want out of life.

A MEDITATION PRIMER

Meditation is simply a means for calming and focusing the searchlight of your awareness so you can directly perceive the super-conscious mind and tap its infinite power. Remember from chapter 3 that the super-conscious mind exists at two levels. The first of these is the individual super-conscious mind—a level of consciousness capable of sensing and influencing the electromagnetic energy fields associated with your body, other people, places, and events—sometimes called the soul. The type of thinking that characterizes individual super-consciousness is intuitive thinking.

The individual super-conscious mind is a portal into an even larger reality, that of universal super-consciousness. Try not to get caught up in the nomenclature here. Call it God, Adonai, Jehovah, Sat, Brahmin, Nirvana, Spirit, or another sacred name based on your religious perspective. The universal super-conscious mind exists as a single quantum (subatomic) intelligent energy field that creates and sustains everything in the universe.

Meditation will allow you to perceive the universal super-conscious mind and your oneness with it. In deep states of meditative thought, you will feel yourself in perfect unity with everything in creation, realize that you and God are one, and understand that you are connected with everyone and everything else in existence. When you gain this awareness, you'll be able to tap its infinite power to heal yourself.

In the last chapter, we used a metaphor to describe this fundamental truth. If you liken the vast sea of super-conscious thought that governs the universe to an ocean, each of us would be like a wave on this ocean—connected into the larger whole, made of the same substance as the ocean. The wave never separates from the ocean. It always has the ocean behind it, sustaining it, and making it go.

Regardless of what you call it, this much is scientifically measurable fact: energy from a source not immediately visible to you sustains you. If you want health and happiness, you need to get in touch with that source. Its very nature is limitless health, compassion, peace, wisdom, love, and joy—the infinite source of every superlative virtue and power. It is in you. You are in it. You *are* it. You are merely unconscious of the fact, and because you are unconscious of it, you cannot tap its power. Meditation will change that in magnificent ways.

It's ironic that we work so hard to attain happiness. We struggle to earn a good living, be healthy, have a wonderful home, a loving family and friends, and a little excitement. Our culture insists that happiness is something you create through activity and effort, and that's understandable on some level, but a very interesting thing happens through meditation—you discover your *basic nature* is happiness. It is (and always has been) inside you at levels so extravagant that nothing in day-to-day experience could quite compare with it. Its nature is "bliss," an ecstatic state of ever-new joy, and with it comes the power and insight you need to heal yourself and accomplish your dreams.

I can't make this point strongly enough: meditation is one of the greatest gifts you will ever receive.

So Many Distractions

Why don't you have this bliss now? I assure you, you are one with the ocean of the universal super-conscious mind—you and God are one. You are simply unaware of it. You are like a corked bottle filled with seawater floating in the ocean. What's keeping the water in that bottle from merging with the ocean? The bottle. If you pop the cork, the bottle sinks and you flow out and merge with the sea around you.

So how do you pop the cork? By getting rid of the distractions confining your awareness. When you stop devoting all your mental energy to the sensory world, you free up that mental energy to focus instead on the ocean of electromagnetic energy behind it. At that point, you will naturally obtain the power to heal yourself.

There are three levels of distraction that keep our awareness "stopped up" in a bottle instead of unified with the ocean of energy around us. The first level consists of the outer distractions: traffic congestion, the weather, IPods, radio, TV, the Xerox machine at the office, the IRS, and even something positive like the birth of a new child in the family. The second level relates to bodily distractions: your backache, your stiff neck, your indigestion, and so forth. Even the effort to breathe and keep your heart beating requires your mental energy (though you may not be consciously aware of it).

Meditation silences these first two levels of distraction by cutting off the "sensory telephones" to the outside world and to the body. This is very different from hypnosis. As we discussed earlier, in hypnosis you remain in touch with the world around you. However, when you meditate deeply, you withdraw the energy that usually flows through your body, to its source in the head—an essential function of good meditative practice called "magnetic pull." You withdraw the energy in your peripheral nerves to the base of the spine and channel it up the spine through the crown of your head where your highest "seat" of awareness is located, your portal to the infinite.

The magnetic pull of meditation has two invaluable benefits. First, as we discussed in chapter 1, if you have no energy in your nerves, you can have no sensory awareness (no electric impulses reach the brain). You may feel as if you do not *have* a body while in a deep meditative state. It's a delightful relief, especially if you suffer from chronic pain. Once you experience the relief, you'll think, "Why didn't I know about this sooner?" Another benefit is that the energy flowing to the crown of your head is now at your disposal to utilize for vast levels of expansion in awareness and power. You can do remarkable things with this energy.

The third level of distraction that keeps us "in a bottle" and unable to tap the power of the ocean is the distraction that comes from the thoughts and feelings in our own minds: that important meeting, the embarrassing situation at work, feeling bad about not showing up at your sister's for Thanksgiving, planning a vacation, gearing up for that parent-teacher conference, remembering to call the doctor, picking up the dry cleaning, and so on. Subconscious fear, sadness, anger, or anxiety also distract and preoccupy our minds.

There's an old saying from the East that dealing with this mental chatter is like trying to tame a wild, drunken monkey. Everyone seeks relief from this chatter at one time or another. The meditation method I'm about to show you will gradually calm these thoughts and feelings until you're left with only pure awareness and profound peace. This is not to say you will enter an unfocused, diffuse state of mind. Meditation will help you achieve perfect mental focus and clarity *and* absolute stillness.

How still can stillness get? Several years ago, I came out of meditation to see a close friend of mine standing directly in front of me, staring at me wide-eyed. As was the case with some of my colleagues, it was her habit to join me for an occasional morning meditation. I asked her what was wrong and she said, "I know I shouldn't have done it Rick, but I opened my eyes while you were meditating and it looked like you weren't breathing. So I got my compact mirror and put it under your nose. Rick—you didn't breathe for twenty-two minutes." I laughed and said, "Yeah, but the important thing is I'm breathing now." I had learned to meditate so deeply, to become so still, that I had no need to burn energy, hence no need for breath. The heart rate and circulation slow measurably during meditation, too. Your body doesn't use energy at these times, so it doesn't need it. Because of this, I have the stamina and vitality of three men, need very little sleep, feel good all the time, am stress-free, and (now that I dealt with that congenital heart problem in my forties) am as healthy as a horse. These benefits of meditation are within reach for everyone who meditates regularly.

THE METHOD

I teach an easy meditation method that has a lot of magnetic pull and has been more thoroughly researched than any other method. To begin, do what you can to limit distractions. Check your bladder, turn off your phone, dim bright lights, and turn off the music. Some people think it's better to meditate with music. Music may make you feel better but it is also a distraction that limits your awareness. You want to have as much silence around you as you reasonably can. Try to find a time to meditate when you won't have to race out the door immediately afterward. At the end of this process, you'll want to maximize the benefits by taking it easy for a few minutes.

Choose a comfortable chair or recliner that allows you to keep your back, neck, and head reasonably aligned and straight (see fig. 7). You don't want to contort your spine because this will impede energy flow. Sitting down is preferable to lying down because the latter invites sleep, but if you have too much discomfort sitting up, by all means, lay down.

Now close your eyes and let your awareness go inward. You want to keep your eyes lifted up slightly under closed lids, as if you were focusing on a far off mountain peak. Neurological studies show that this position of the eyes encourages peace (if the eyes are looking straight ahead, you'll "think" a lot; whereas, if you lower your eyes, you might get sleepy).

If you are a person of faith, this would be a good time to engage in a brief prayer or invocation for guidance.

Start the meditative process by monitoring your breathing. Don't time or control it. You are not trying to harness your breath in any way. Just let it go in and out on its own. Breathe in at the point you find the body breathing in. Breathe out at the point you find the body breathing out. It doesn't matter if it's slow and deep or rapid and shallow. Let the breath do whatever it wants, but observe it closely. If you're a beginner, do this for about three minutes while not allowing any other thought to distract you. If something does distract you, (a sound, a feeling in your body, or a concern, for example), gently return your attention to your breath as it flows in and out.

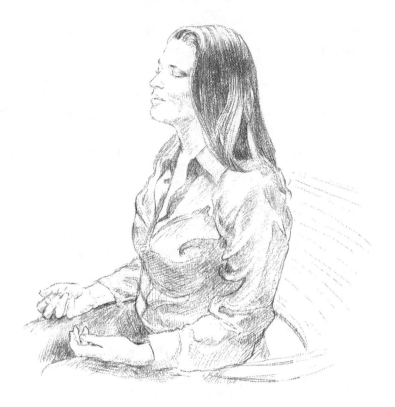

FIGURE 7

Next, for the length of the out-breath only, mentally say to yourself the word "*Om*" (pronounced *awm*). *Om* is a remarkable sound. EEG studies have demonstrated that silent repetition of *Om* causes brain waves to become very relaxed and smooth out while increasing mental clarity. *Om* is actually the sound of super-consciousness, the "hum" of intelligent energy, all the sounds of the universe in one. The silent chanting of *Om* on the out-breath will significantly calm and focus your mind, removing distractions.

If you are a beginner, try observing the breath and silently saying *Om* on the out-breath for at least five minutes. In all likelihood, you're going to drift off into a thought, a feeling, a daydream, or an anticipation of some sort. At first, you may not even realize you've drifted off. After all, it's perfectly normal for one's thoughts to wander. As soon as you realize it, however, let go of what you're thinking or feeling and come back to the method: *Om* on the out-breath.

You will gradually drift off less and less. Think of a glass jar filled with mud and water. If you shake it and put it on a table, at first you'll see a million specks whirling about. Those specks are like all the thoughts and feelings moving through you. As you let the jar sit on the table, though, allowing it to achieve stillness, you'll see the specks settle down until the water above the mud becomes crystal clear. If you meditate every day, you'll find that thought and reactive emotion will settle down and stop completely. At that point, your mind becomes like the clear water in the jar. You will then naturally experience your own super-conscious mind—a level of awareness that exists behind your everyday thoughts and feelings.

You cannot stop "thinking" as an act of will. Instead, you'll be busy thinking about not thinking. The method is the key here—silent chanting of *Om* with the out-breath. By returning to the method each time you drift off, you'll start locating your consciousness in a place that is "outside" of thought and feeling altogether. This is also your point of access into the universal super-conscious mind. When your mind is like the crystal-clear water in the jar, then you can stop the method (no focus on the breath, no *Om* on the out-breath). Now it's time to sit in the stillness and simply dwell in the extravagant joy, peace, and power of the super-conscious mind.

Even before you arrive fully at this destination, if you keep meditating, you will inherit the benefits right away—both in and *out* of meditation. The first thing you will notice is peace, the kind of tranquility that keeps deepening into joy. Optimism and confidence will rise naturally. You will feel physically better right away and keep improving: less pain, more mobility. You will also start to develop intuitive wisdom (for example, you will just *know* which doctor to go to, which diet is best, which medication to choose, whether to have surgery now or wait).

Early in meditation, you will actually begin to feel *larger* because meditation increases the size of your electromagnetic energy field. With that increase comes much greater awareness and power. You will start sensing and directing the energy fields associated with yourself as well as other people, places, and events. You may begin to intuit how other people feel, sense the intelligence in the plants in your garden for the first time, or even have a foreknowledge of future events and be able to shift them with your thoughts.

If you stay with meditation, you will also begin to notice that the things you need are being drawn to you—the right medical specialist, a big raise just when the medical bills are piling up, and so on. Just as important, your own nature will become transparent to you. Your *story behind the story* will emerge and you will have the power to change it or keep it as you desire. It will seem to you that life doesn't get any better, but it does. Keep meditating, and life will keep getting better and better.

HYPNOTICALLY GUIDED MEDITATION

You can meditate on your own using the simple method I've just described, or you can allow me to assist you. You know from your work in previous chapters that hypnosis is an extremely powerful tool for calming the body and mind. When you first start meditating, you may find that you cannot relax or that your thoughts drift off with such frequency that you have trouble getting to a meditative state. I have developed a hypnotic process to help you overcome these challenges quickly and bring you to the clear, focused mind needed for effective meditation.

For this hypnotic assist with your meditation, download Induction Alpha-III from www.miraculoushealthbook.com and burn it onto a CD. Set aside some time and prepare yourself just as if you were going to meditate on your own (check your bladder, limit the distractions, dim bright lights, and situate yourself comfortably with spine and head aligned). Now start the download. In it, I will use a progressive relaxation induction and guided imagery to calm your mind and body and then walk you through the meditation method. From that point onward, I will leave you to meditate for twenty minutes before emerging you from the process.

YOUR PLAN FOR DEVELOPING SKILL IN MEDITATION

Whether you choose to meditate on your own or rely on a hypnotic assist, start meditating now. The first day you meditate, and for a few days thereafter, try meditating for just ten minutes. If you find you've drifted off onto a thought or feeling (this happens to everyone from time to time), simply come back to the method. Some beginning meditators have trouble with intrusive thoughts and feelings and believe they *can't* meditate. This is absolutely not true. Just stick with the method, and you'll be delighted with the results.

After the first few days, let the time you spend meditating expand naturally. Many of us are so problem-focused and achievement-oriented that we'll turn anything into a job. It isn't necessary to make meditation another one. Try for those ten minutes and anything you can do thereafter. The experience will grow naturally and in a pleasant way. If you stick with the process, you'll soon find yourself spending an hour or more in daily meditation, just because you enjoy its benefits so much.

Continue to practice meditation as you move forward through subsequent chapters. Strive to meditate at least three times per week because regular meditation will serve as a foundation for your success no matter what your personal goals for self-healing. The health effects of long-term daily meditation are dramatic. For now, though, you've given yourself a tremendous gift. This simple procedure will help you feel measurably better right away.

YOUR TOOL BELT IS COMPLETE

You now have the three tools you need to move effectively through the rest of our process:

- *Feeling Energy.* You have learned to:
  * Create an energy bubble.
  * Use the bubble to move energy to various parts of the body.
  * Use your hands to feel the energy in a partner.
  * Perform an internal tour of your energies.
  * Use your body to feel the energy in others.
- *Hypnosis.* You have learned to:
  * Experience hypnosis.
  * Feel energy while in a hypnotic state.
- *Meditation.* You have learned to:
  * Experience meditation.
  * Use hypnosis to augment the meditation experience.

Practice these methods for the suggested ten-day period before you move on to the next section of the book. The great thing about the work you're doing here is that all of it has an immediate benefit. Each of these tools will improve your sense of health and wellbeing right away. The remarkable thing is that we haven't even begun to utilize them for analysis and treatment. The sense of wonder, peace, and physical satisfaction you gain during this initial phase is considerable, and you should enjoy it and have fun with it.

Remember, this is only the beginning. What comes after this is exponentially more miraculous.

PART TWO

SELF-ANALYSIS

CHAPTER 5

CONSCIOUS ASSESSMENT

N ow that you've learned the basic skills you need to get the most out of this program, it's time to begin exploring the mental causes that have been fueling your health concerns. In this chapter, I'll walk you through a process that will help you begin to understand your *story behind the story.* You'll need this understanding to take advantage of the tools provided in this book—tools that will allow you to free yourself from your past and move into a future of health and happiness.

Let's start by reiterating two powerful principles from chapter 1.

First, every disease in the body begins with dis-ease in the mind. There is a mental root for every physical problem. If you discover this root and heal it, your physical health will improve. There are no exceptions. Remember Erin's story and my story? Even if your health problem is congenital or hereditary, the result of an accident, or the result of environmental factors (such as an exposure to a toxic chemical), you can dramatically improve your health if you discover the mental root that caused the health problem to take hold.

Second, living outside your *story*—not learning the lessons that life is trying to teach you, misunderstanding or repressing your experience, or living a life that is inauthentic to your highest desires—is the root cause of physical suffering. I'm not suggesting you brought your physical issues onto yourself. Very few people can understand what life is trying to tell them. Life is complicated and many of us are not empowered with the tools needed to understand and navigate it. I wrote this book to help you with this, and this chapter will aid you by helping you understand your *story* more deeply and authentically than you have before.

In subsequent chapters, I'll help you "mine" your *story* for its deepest insights, as well as for its beauty—every person's life is a noble, epic adventure in self-understanding, even if the circumstances have been difficult. Later, I will show you how to delve very deeply into the meaning of your life. I will also show you how to change your *story* if you desire, but for now, start by trying to understand it as a history, with an eye toward where it's leading you.

WHERE ARE YOU RIGHT NOW?

We'll begin with a simple conscious assessment (what you are aware of right now) of your *story*. The process I describe here will help you understand:

- The major twists and turns of your life, how they've affected you, how you've reacted to them, and the extent to which they've confined or liberated you.
- How well you've fared so far relative to your expectations.
- The major themes threading through your experience and what they imply about who you are and where you're going.

We'll use an effective "broad brush" approach to conduct our conscious assessment, similar to what a therapist does during the first session or two with a new client. We're going to keep it simple, using a qualitative approach that relies on short narrative accounts, a brief series of self-rating scales, and answers to a few short questions. All you'll need is a pad of paper or a computer and some time set aside to consider the texture of your life. Then, answer the following questions with as much honesty as you can muster and at a pace you find comfortable. You can always return to one or more questions after you've finished the assessment.

1. WHO ARE THE FIVE PEOPLE WHO'VE HAD THE BIGGEST INFLUENCE ON YOU?

Go back as far as you can remember. List each name and write a sentence or two explaining why you've chosen this person. Keep going beyond five if you can think of more, but remember that these are the people who have had *the biggest influence on your life.* Be sure to list people who've had a negative influence, not just the mentors and saviors.

2. WHAT ARE THE FIVE MAJOR EVENTS THAT HAVE SHAPED YOUR LIFE?

The key here is to identify the events that have had the greatest impact on you, whether pro or con. Again, go back in time as far as you can remember. Write down each event and a sentence about why it was important. Remember subtle but powerful events like falling in love for the first time or the birth of a child. Be sure to consider events that have had an impact on you from a cultural or world perspective, such as Martin Luther King's "I Have a Dream" speech, the fall of the Berlin Wall, the emergence of the internet, and so on. If you can think of more than five life-changing events, write them down.

3. WHAT REALLY JAZZES YOU IN LIFE?

Give this careful thought and write detailed answers. Has a particular passion had an important place in your world for as long as you can remember? Do you love dancing, sports, travel, or community service? Is there a cause that moves you or a specific philosophical, political, or religious theme that underscores your outlook on life? Can you notice repetitive patterns of attachment to a cause or a particular way of being? How might your interests have changed over time, and why? For example, you may have had a long-standing love of medicine and entered nursing school but dropped out to have children and never went back.

Try to synthesize the aspects of your history as they relate to "what really jazzes you in life" and then sum them up as a metaphor(s) for who you really are. For example, at heart you may be a healer, warrior, lover, sage, statesman, mother, caregiver, musician, artist, writer, public servant, entrepreneur, saint, or something else.

4. WRITE DOWN YOUR LIFE SCRIPT.

Write down your history in two or three pages, as if you were writing the synopsis to the Hollywood screenplay of your life. Do it in chronological order: birthplace, family of origin, schools, moves, jobs, important relationships, memorable accomplishments, major setbacks, lost love, births of children, and so on. Chronicle the five major people (question 1) and five major events at the point they occurred (question 2), along with important events relating to the things that jazz you (question 3). Be sure to write down approximate dates for the onset of your illness, changes in your health over time, and relevant medical information regarding diagnosis, treatment, and prognosis for your medical condition(s).

5. RATE YOURSELF ACCORDING TO EACH OF THE FOLLOWING SCALES.

What follows is a series of highly personal and subjective self-rating scales. I've designed them to provide you with a snapshot of where you are. These will help you develop a plan for growth and provide a baseline against which you can measure your future progress. These scales are *not* quantitative, scientifically validated psychometric testing methods, and this is intentional. This means *I'm* not scoring you; *you* are. The intent of these scores is not to compare them with anyone else's. For example, one of the scales asks you to rate how successful you've been in your major life role. A successful mother of three children may rate herself at one (the best score) on a scale of one to seven. A successful NASA rocket scientist may also rate herself at one, but the results would be strictly non-comparable.

Now score yourself using the following twelve scales. Rate yourself based on your own attitudes, expectations, thoughts, and feelings. These are seven-point scales—a rating of one is the best outcome and a seven the worst. We used ten-point scales to assess your physical pain in previous chapters because that is the standard in use among most hospitals and healthcare settings in the United States. We're using seven-point scales in this chapter because they are simpler and just as effective for self-assessment purposes.

Rate yourself by circling the number that represents your self-assessment. Be sure to read the guidelines provided for each scale.

5A. HOW AWARE ARE YOU?

1 * 2 * 3 * 4 * 5 * 6 * 7

How present are you to what is going on in your environment, body, and mind? A rating of one indicates you are immediately aware of changes in your health, your mental state, and the world around you. A rating of seven indicates a profound lack of awareness regarding all three. You'll want to consider your general level of awareness as you move through the remaining scales.

5B. HOW SERIOUS ARE YOUR HEALTHCARE CONCERNS?

1 * 2 * 3 * 4 * 5 * 6 * 7

Rate how serious your problem is, one being the least serious and seven being a major life-threatening condition, such as cancer.

5C. HOW MOBILE AND FUNCTIONAL IS YOUR BODY?

1 * 2 * 3 * 4 * 5 * 6 * 7

Rate your body's overall level of mobility and functioning. A one indicates outstanding mobility and functioning (no one can even tell you are ill), and a seven indicates little or no mobility and/or functionality. Rate yourself without the use of physical aids (a wheelchair, cane, or orthotic device, for example).

5D. RATE YOUR PAIN.

1 * 2 * 3 * 4 * 5 * 6 * 7

Rate your pain on a scale of one to seven, with one being no pain at all and seven being the worst pain you can imagine.

5E. HOW HAPPY AND JOYFUL DO YOU FEEL?

1 * 2 * 3 * 4 * 5 * 6 * 7

A rating of one on this scale means you're happy and joyful all the time, and a seven means you are unhappy almost all the time.

5F. HOW SUCCESSFUL ARE YOU IN YOUR MAJOR LIFE ROLE?

1 * 2 * 3 * 4 * 5 * 6 * 7

Measure your success relative to your most important role in life as you define it. The question is equally applicable to the CEO of a major corporation as for a stay-at-home mom. If you feel strongly that you have two equally important roles in life (say that of being a great husband and that of being a successful entrepreneur), then scale your progress in both roles.

5G. HOW MUCH MEANING AND PURPOSE DO YOU GET OUT OF LIFE?

1 * 2 * 3 * 4 * 5 * 6 * 7

Define meaning and purpose in whatever way works best for you, then scale your status. A rating of one means your life is abundant with meaning and purpose, and a seven means you feel a total vacuum of meaning and purpose in life.

5H. HOW GOOD ARE YOUR MOST IMPORTANT RELATIONSHIPS?

1 * 2 * 3 * 4 * 5 * 6 * 7

Consider the strength of your relationships with family, friends, colleagues, and lovers. A rating of one indicates your relationships are, by and large, mutually supportive and highly rewarding, while a seven indicates your relationships are, by and large, harmful.

5I. HOW WELL DO YOU LIKE YOURSELF?

1 * 2 * 3 * 4 * 5 * 6 * 7

This is a self-acceptance scale. A rating of one indicates you respect yourself and are very happy with who you are. A rating of seven indicates you have no self-acceptance whatsoever (you can't stand yourself).

5J. HOW GOOD IS THE LOVE IN YOUR LIFE?

1 * 2 * 3 * 4 * 5 * 6 * 7

A rating of one indicates a life rich in love from any number of sources: girlfriend or boyfriend, spouse, family members, friends, a family of faith, associates. You can be single and still feel richly loved. A rating of seven means you have no love in your life whatsoever.

5K. HOW WOULD YOU RATE YOUR OVERALL PERSONAL GROWTH?

1 * 2 * 3 * 4 * 5 * 6 * 7

A rating of one indicates you're extremely satisfied with your rate of personal growth (you've been continually making progress despite obstacles), and a rating of seven indicates you are extremely dissatisfied (no personal growth at all).

5L. HOW DIFFICULT DO YOU THINK YOUR LIFE HAS BEEN SO FAR?

1 * 2 * 3 * 4 * 5 * 6 * 7

A rating of one indicates you've had a great life (no complaints). A rating of seven indicates you've had the worst possible life story (if it hadn't been for bad luck, you wouldn't have any luck at all).

6. DEVELOP A LIST OF STRENGTHS AND CHALLENGES.

Go back to questions 1 through 5 and review your assessment so far. Be sure to look at the big picture, as well as the trends and details, and be sure to analyze your answers to the scales in question 5, as they will provide you with very keen insight into the texture of your story.

Now sit down with a piece of paper and draw a line down the middle from top to bottom. At the top of the left column write "Strengths" and at the top of the right column write "Challenges."

Start with your strengths. Keep going until you've identified at least five. They should leap out of your assessment. For example, perhaps your life has been very difficult (scale 5b) and your physical pain very high (scale 5d), but you consider yourself happy (scale 5e) and are making good personal progress despite your difficulties (scale 5k). That's extraordinary, and you need to explain why that is. Perhaps you are strong-willed, courageous, and innately optimistic, or maybe, you are a person of deep faith. Whatever it is, write it down in the strengths column. Even if your assessment paints a despairing picture, you will still be able to identify at least five strengths. You are a survivor. Ask yourself why that is so, and write down the strengths that have enabled you to persevere.

After you've finished your list of strengths (which you can always return to later), move on to your challenges. These will also leap off the pages of your assessment. Is lack of awareness something that has complicated your life? Has it caused you to lose in love or otherwise miss opportunities to fulfill your dreams? If so, improving your awareness is a challenge. Write it down. Perhaps you are alone and overly alienated from other people. Why? Or perhaps you need to develop more self-acceptance. If so, you'll want to identify what stands between you and better self-love and respect. Write down at least five challenges you can identify. Do the best you can. You can return to this list later after you've made gains in self-understanding. At some point you'll want to refine the list and/or prioritize your challenges in order of most important to least.

7. HOW WELL HAVE YOU LIVED OUT YOUR STORY SO FAR?

Given the results of your assessment, how would you rate your performance as the lead character in the story of your life? Rate yourself on the following scale.

1 * 2 * 3 * 4 * 5 * 6 * 7

A rating of one signifies you think you've done a great job moving through your life given what you had on your plate. A rating of seven means you'd give anything to have the chance to go back and do it differently.

TIME TO LOOK DEEPER

I want you to take time now to appreciate the uniqueness of your story and its beauty. No matter how you answered question 7, I assure you that if you had to go back and live your story out again with only the knowledge you had at the time, you'd live it out precisely the way you have. There's nobility in that—regardless of how you feel about your life. You've learned things you would not have learned otherwise and accomplished what was important to you and those you love. There is greatness in you and in your story, and there's a very good chance this has escaped your attention. Physical or emotional pain or past trauma might be obscuring it for you, but it is there if you know how to see it.

Some years ago, a beautiful young woman in her early thirties came to see me. She suffered from severe dysmenorrhea (painful menstruation) and stomach ulcers, neither of which responded to medical treatment. Her history was remarkable for early childhood trauma: her dad was an abusive alcoholic. He berated her often, and though he never actually raped her, he was guilty of behavioral incest—he would touch her inappropriately in intimate ways and sometimes crawl into bed with her at night. She grew up in constant terror but placated him out of loyalty to her younger siblings whom she strove to protect from her father. She left home at eighteen and worked as a waitress at night in addition to odd day jobs to put herself through college. She was devoted to God and to human welfare. She seemed to me to be very pure of heart. Still, though outwardly calm and sophisticated, she carried enough anxiety around with her to sink the Titanic.

During our first session, she said, "I have a confession to make ... the worst thing I've ever done ... I've never told it to anyone." She went on to say that, while a junior in college, she entered a contest for "Centerfold Campus Coed." She won and very briefly embarked on a career as a nude centerfold model. "The money was so good and I was desperate, so I did it." Unfortunately, she had never been able to live with the guilt this experience caused her. She felt dreadful about this and carried it as another burden.

I saw nothing but beauty in her story. Her anxiety had been perpetrated on her by her father and was quite literally "eating away at her" in the form of her stomach ulcers. His sexual misconduct combined with abuse had stolen her self-esteem and caused her to see her sexuality as the source of fear and shame. This mental dis-ease lodged in her reproductive organs, hence the dysmenorrhea.

During the course of our work together, which involved talk therapy and hypnosis to release the fear, shame, and guilt she carried, she began to embrace her own nobility—her devotion to her siblings under extreme duress, the courage and discipline demonstrated after being banished from home, her dogged insistence on a bright future, her compassion for others, and her faith. She even came to understand how her nude modeling was a natural offshoot of her powerfully negative experience with her own sexuality.

She shifted away from anxiety and into self-love and even began to glimpse the high regard with which she was held in the mind of God. The ulcers and the dysmenorrhea went away, and she became truly happy.

I served as this woman's ally in the process, but you can do this for yourself with the methods I provide in this book. The assessment you're doing in this chapter is an extremely valuable step, one that will help you consider your *story behind the story*. It will help you see the nobility in the life you've lived so far.

It is possible to find beauty or ugliness in anything you look at or anything you experience. If you look closely enough at a painting by a great master, you'll find some of the brush strokes aren't quite right. If you focus on what's negative, that's what you'll see. If, instead, you think of your life as an epic adventure in self-discovery with you as its hero, you'll see something else entirely. Something inspirational and affirming. Something to drive you to higher levels. Why not start right now?

I want you to step entirely outside your life and look at it as though you are reading a novel or watching a movie. Find the audience appeal in your story. See the triumphs and losses, the joys and betrayals, and great breaks and the missed opportunities as part of a heroic saga that has an underlying purpose. Ask yourself:

- What are the major themes in this saga?
- What is the central mission of the hero (you)?
- What are your strengths? How has the "screenplay" hidden these strengths or brought them to light?
- What are your flaws? How does the "action" challenge you to overcome these flaws?
- Who are the "bad guys" and other antagonists that confront you on your mission? How do you deal with them?
- What would constitute justice for you, and how do you go about getting it?
- When and how are you aided on your quest? When will the cavalry come over the hill (there's always a cavalry, and you might be it)?

Look closely for metaphorical and symbolic meaning: did the hero break his back after he tried to carry the weight of the world on his shoulders by working two jobs to support his family? Did she develop congestive heart failure after a string of lost loves in her life?

Take out a piece of paper and write down the most essential things you can appreciate about your life as an epic journey in self-discovery, about you as hero. You are beginning to see the *story behind the story*. I will help you explore this in greater depth in subsequent chapters.

START TO LOOK AHEAD

Now is the time to begin thinking about how you want the story to continue. You are in fact the screenwriter of your own destiny and can dictate where the story will go from here. I'm going to show you how.

Your true adventure with my methods is only beginning. This assessment will present you with an image of yourself that you've likely never seen before. It will move you in unexpected ways. It will open new doors for you.

And there's even more to discover.

CHAPTER 6

HYPNOTIC SELF-ASSESSMENT

I n this chapter, we will use hypnosis to help you understand more about the relationship between illness in your body and your *story behind the story*. The process will involve scanning your body, identifying places where you have some level of discomfort or dysfunction, and "inquiring" as to the underlying mental cause—all while you are under hypnosis.

In order to do this effectively though, you need to have a better understanding of energy centers in the body and the symbolic presentation of disease.

ENERGY CENTERS IN THE BODY

You have a body of energy that sustains your physical body: the BioEM energy field we've explored in previous chapters. Your "energy body" exists within your physical body and expands outward from it. However, within the body it "mirrors" your physical structure. The BioEM energy body contains a series of "energy centers" located in the spine and head. If you have practiced the methods in chapter 2, you might already sense these energy centers in yourself or others.

Energy healers are keenly aware of the location and significance of energy centers in the BioEM energy field. Since your health is important to you, awareness of these energy centers will prove invaluable in your quest toward improved wellbeing.

There are many medical models for understanding how energy flows through the body. In the West, modern neuroscience describes the movement of energy from the brain, down the spine, through the peripheral nervous system, and then from the extremities back to the spine and brain through a series of nerve centers or "bundles and branches" (energy centers) in the spine. Chinese medicine describes the flow of energy from the brain through the body in a series of meridians, or energy pathways, as well as areas in the body where energy ("chi") is concentrated. The rishis of India developed a scheme of bodily energy flow based on chakras. Chakra is Sanskrit for "wheel," and Hindu medicine describes a series of distinct energy centers (spinning wheels of concentrated energy) in the head, spine, and to a lesser degree, in the extremities. Well-trained energy healers see the chakras with their physical eyes, and the chakras do in fact appear as whirling wheels or vortices of light and color.

All these schemes have a commonality: energy flows from the brain outward into the peripheral nervous system and back again, and there are places in the body where energy is concentrated. The flow of energy in a robust, unimpeded, and positive way throughout the system assures bodily health. However, if the energy flow through the body is sluggish, blocked, dampened, or negative in one or more energy centers, then health is poor.

In the hypnotic exercise at the conclusion of this chapter, I will escort you through an internal diagnostic of your bodily energies. Remember, energy in the body follows thought. As we move through important energy centers in your body under hypnosis, you will explore the "thought" or the *story behind the story* that will help explain why you hold energy the way you do, where you do. You will be able to diagnose the mental root behind your dis-ease in different energy centers of the body. In short, you will put another significant piece of your health puzzle in place.

The first energy center is at the very bottom of the spine between the legs (see fig. 8). This energy center stores basic biological energy. It's like a battery responsible for fueling the body. A person who lacks sufficient energy here or who holds a lot of negative energy in this center will feel drained and weakened, as though his gas tank is always running on empty. This person will get sick often and be especially prone to infectious diseases, such as colds or the flu.

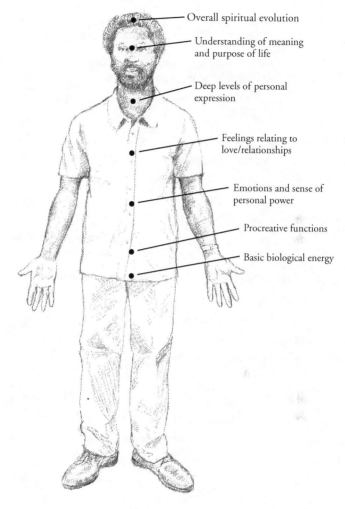

Overall spiritual evolution

Understanding of meaning
and purpose of life

Deep levels of personal
expression

Feelings relating to
love/relationships

Emotions and sense of
personal power

Procreative functions

Basic biological energy

FIGURE 8

A second, important energy center exists in the area of the genitals. This center fuels your procreative functions. A person who lacks sufficient energy here or chronically stores a lot of negative energy in this center might suffer from impotence or infertility or be prone to disorders of the reproductive organs: dysmenorrhea, endometriosis, prostate dysfunction or cancer, fibroid tumors in women, or even cancer of the vagina, cervix, or uterus.

A third, important energy center encompasses the digestive system, pancreas, and liver. This is where we store emotion and hold our sense of personal power. When people have problems in this energy center, they often manifest as eating disorders, intestinal disorders, or diseases of the pancreas or liver.

The fourth energy center surrounds the heart. This is where we store energies and emotions relating to love, family relationships, and long-term friendships. The heart is also a center for human virtue (honesty, loyalty, trustworthiness, courage, and so forth). As we've already discussed, when people have problems in this energy center, they tend to show up as heart disease or pulmonary problems.

The fifth energy center is in the throat. This center is where we hold energies, thoughts, and feelings associated with deep levels of personal expression—our ability to address what matters most. People who are very good communicators usually have very strong energy in the throat center. By contrast, people who withhold expression have weak or negative energy in this center and tend to suffer from disorders like chronic laryngitis.

The sixth energy center is in the head. This is where we store our understanding of meaning and purpose in life. When the energies in the head are strong and healthy, the person is powerfully in touch with his or her *story behind the story.*

The energy flow through the head has two poles: the point between the eyebrows (the third eye) and the medullar center (the area at the back of the head where the head meets the spine, adjacent to the medulla oblongata, or brainstem). The medullar center is a portal through which energy from the super-conscious mind flows into the body. In the New Testament, Jesus says, "Man does not live by bread alone but by every word that proceedeth forth from the mouth of God." "The mouth of God" is a metaphor for the medullar center, and "word" is a metaphor for universal life force (the Holy Spirit). Jesus was trying to tell his followers the life force in the body is a function of universal super-conscious energy flow through the medullar center and not simply a function of the energy ingested through food. The medullar sub-energy center is very sensitive and can be blocked easily by stress, physical trauma, and negative emotional energies.

From the medullar center, energy flows in two directions: down to the base of the spine to help power the body and forward through the brain to the forehead, or third eye. The medullar center acts as a battery that energetically fuels both the body and our higher awareness. For the same reason, the point between the eyebrows is a place where intuitive insight is sharp.

Because the head is "command central" for the entire nervous system, when the energies in the head are low, congested, or negative, the brain and nervous system are at-risk. People who chronically hold negative energy in this center are prone to migraines, stroke, cancer, or disorders of the central nervous system. They may also suffer from chronic sinus, ear, and eye problems.

The seventh energy center is at the very top of the head. This center has to do with the overall spiritual evolution of a person. It does not necessarily tell you the merit of the individual, however. A fine, virtuous person whom you admire might not be particularly evolved spiritually while someone who is highly evolved might be letting all of that spiritual power go to waste. When the energies in this center are strong, you might feel a deep sense of connection to something larger than yourself and experience strong intuitive awareness. When they are weak, you may feel like an island, set off from other people and the world around you.

SYMBOLIC PRESENTATION

As you now know, every disease or injury in the body has a mental root—some form of dis-ease in your thought and feeling. This mental dis-ease exists in the BioEM field as subtle electromagnetic energy, and the subconscious mind tends to symbolically place these subtle mental energies in the body. For instance:

- A person might have shoulder problems because she's "shouldering a burden" or feels "the weight of the world on her shoulders."
- Someone with diabetes might have trouble digesting the "sweetness" of life; he has no time to stop and smell the roses because he's too busy conquering the world.
- A person with neck problems may feel as if she is constantly "sticking her neck out" and taking too many risks, or perhaps her basic attitude about life is that most of it is "a pain in the neck."
- Someone with problems in his hands might have trouble "getting a hold" of life.
- People with heart problems have often suffered too much loss of love.

- Problems with the feet tend to indicate that a person has trouble feeling grounded in the world; she just doesn't feel comfortable standing on terra firma.
- Those with joint problems tend to be people who block their emotions; their emotional inflexibility moves to the joints and they become physically rigid.
- People who have trouble with their vision tend to be blocking or holding back something important in their lives that they don't want to see.
- In the same way, those with poor hearing tend to have something they don't want to hear.
- People who have problems with their mouths, jaws, or throat tend to hold back meaningful self-expression—literally "choking" on words unsaid.
- Lower back problems have to do with power and control issues—how we gird our lower back to "heft" the demands of life.

In most cases, the subconscious mind's "symbolic" way of lodging illness in the body is obvious. There's a good reason for this: disease is symbolically placed to communicate to the conscious mind that mental dis-ease or disharmony requires attention. This is a clarion call. The subconscious mind does not mean to harm us. Rather, it seeks to alert us to a problem and get us back on track. Consider this as you move through the hypnotic assessment at the end of this chapter.

INTERRELATEDNESS

Because of the way energy flows in the body, the energy centers are in constant communication with each other. Dis-ease in one energy center fuels problems in others.

A middle-aged woman named Joan came to me two years ago with complaints of severe pain in her lumbar spine. She was an avid horseback rider who owned a farm, stables, and horses. She'd been on the competitive riding circuit for years until the pain in her spine became so acute she could no longer ride. By the time she got to me, she was severely depressed over the loss of her life's ambition. Things were so bad from her perspective that she just wanted to die. Her orthopedist had diagnosed her problem as degenerative disc disease—its onset undoubtedly due to the concussions to her spine she'd endured while riding. He told her the only answer was surgery and said there was a good chance she'd never ride again.

The cause the orthopedist suggested makes sense, but at the same time, many career riders never develop severe spine problems. Obviously, the key to Joan's dilemma was in her *story behind the story*. I did an energy diagnostic on Joan and picked up a lot of negativity in the third energy center (the stomach and lumbar spine). She carried a great deal of pain and anxiety there. The medullar energy center at the base of her head was partially blocked—very little energy was flowing through it because the anxiety she carried in her stomach and lower back was channeling up her spine and "blocking up" this sensitive center. There was a lot of negative energy concentrated in her throat, indicating she was choking back some powerful emotion.

I asked her some questions about her life. She and her husband lived on their farm. He was a very prominent man, whose work regularly took him away from home, leaving the chores to Joan. Meanwhile, Joan had a retail business to run in addition to managing the farm and horses. She had a demanding mother and an equally demanding mother-in-law living with her. She also had a child with emotional issues. On top of this, Joan was a perfectionist and wanted everything done right. There was simply no way she could handle everything she "carried on her back," which eventually broke under the weight of her responsibilities.

I did energy work on Joan's spine to provide immediate relief from pain and begin the healing of her body. To get to the underlying cause of her problem, we used hypnosis and cathartic release techniques (you'll learn more about these in a short while) to free her from pent-up anxiety. She relied on hypnotically guided meditation to reduce her stress. Throughout, I taught her to take a different approach toward life, letting others take more responsibility for their welfare. I told her, "If God wanted you to be a beast of burden you'd have been born a donkey." She heard me and learned to take it a little easier. She found her voice and recovered from her depression. Together with her husband, they moved their mothers off the farm. Her back healed, and she could ride again. Her outlook on life improved enormously.

HYPNOTIC SELF-ASSESSMENT

Before you start the hypnotic self-assessment, take a little time to review the results of your work from chapter 2 (especially exercise 4: Feeling Energy Internally), chapter 3 (hypnotic assessment of energy in the body), and chapter 5 (conscious assessment). This brief review will give you important reference points for the work you're going to do next and improve the results.

With the hypnotic self-assessment, you'll discover the relationship between your bodily energies and your *story behind the story*. For example, let's say that you felt unease in your heart during exercise 4 and the hypnotic energy assessment. Your doctor has diagnosed you with plaque in the arteries of your heart, for which you take medication. Your autobiography touches on the difficult relationship with your mother, who was never fully emotionally available to you. Perhaps you forgave her and went on with life, and you think the story ended there. Then you go into hypnosis.

When you scan your heart under hypnosis, you discover the relationship with your mother caused more pain than you've been willing to admit and that you've been blocking it. Your heart feels tight, straining against its walls like there's a fortress around it. A picture of your mother's face might flash into your mind as you focus on this tight feeling. You'll see that the dynamic with your mother affected your dating life when you got older. Sometimes you were callous and gruff to romantic partners. You found a way to deal with this and became a little more open and caring, but you're surprised to experience how much pain you still carry, how much you still hold back. With stark clarity, you realize this pain is standing in the way of a more openhearted relationship with your wife. These are huge and important revelations.

The door to the subconscious mind is open during hypnosis, and as you contemplate any pain you might feel in a focused way, it may offer you symbols or images that provide you with greater insight. You may see a picture of a broken heart or a heart in a prison or see yourself living on an island in isolation. You can see quite clearly that this symbolic approach to life has had an enormously negative impact on your physical health.

The door to the super-conscious mind is also open during your hypnotic assessment. You might recollect how you were as a child, filled with exuberance and optimism and delighted with the simple joys of life. It might dawn on you that this is your true nature. Then you realize the pain you carry in your heart limits your natural zeal for life, your search for meaning, and other things you used to hold dear but lost long ago. You would see with profound clarity that your lessons have to do with healing the old pain and calling out the deeper, better part of you so you can live the most successful, joyful life imaginable. It isn't necessary for you to be an island. You are innately loving and optimistic. You begin to see a need for reclaiming your highest nature. Again, these are huge discoveries. They're not only possible during the hypnotic assessment—they're *likely*.

When you do this scan under hypnosis, you might see any number of relationships between your physical problems and the degree of mental disease you carry. This will lead you to tremendous revelation. Explore this openly, and you'll come away from this process with a collection of valuable insights that will give you a huge amount of power over your wellbeing. This type of experience usually carries with it a sense of adventurous awe, as Christopher Columbus felt when he sighted the West Indies for the first time—a sense of "Eureka, I found it." In any event, know that whatever disease you may uncover during this process, I'll provide you with the means to heal it in the remainder of this book so you can go on to live the life you were born to live. You're doing yourself a great deal of good by going on this "exploration."

To do the hypnotic self-assessment, download Induction Beta-I from www.miraculoushealthbook.com and burn it to a CD. Then set up the room for privacy and silence as you have for the other hypnotic exercises. Now play the CD. In it, I will take you into hypnosis and then on a guided tour of the energy centers in your body.

You will want to keep track of your observations during the process. You can do this in one of two ways; either have a pad of paper and pen nearby to write down your insights or set up a tape recorder for the observations you will speak aloud during the process (you can go back to the tape later for review or even transcribe the recording onto paper).

If you decide to write down your observations, you'll remain fully under hypnosis while you're writing. Though I've introduced you to hypnosis in a relaxed quiet setting, there are many times when I hypnotize clients while they are out in their own worlds. For instance, if I were using hypnosis to help you become a better worker, I'd have you in a hypnotic state while you were working in your office. As I guide you through the hypnotic assessment, I will stop at intervals and invite you to write or speak about your observations. Then I'll return you to a deep hypnotic state after each pause in the process. You won't lose anything.

THE STORY BEHIND THE STORY REVEALED

At the end of this process, you will have amassed a substantial amount of information—your conscious assessment from chapter 5 and the hypnotic self-assessment you just completed. You now have an incredibly deep and valuable analysis that speaks volumes about your own *story behind the story*. You're very close to uncovering the root cause of the mental dis-ease responsible for your physical ill health.

It's time to write your story. Before you start, though, let me caution you about two things. First, avoid the "medical student syndrome." In medical school, young doctors-to-be studying symptoms and illness will often conclude they have a disease themselves just because they carry a few of its symptoms. Make sure you are authoring your own story and not someone else's. You've read many stories in this book. Your story, however, is unique. Among billions of people in the world, there is only one you. Look deeply into the texture of your life to find your own unique story.

The second caution concerns the human tendency to evaluate one's life against the accomplishments or expectations of other people. When it comes down to deriving an accurate, honest understanding of your story, you want to be careful not to make unrealistic comparisons to others. Ram Dass once told a story that is relevant here. Remember, he came from a very wealthy family and therefore associated with other wealthy people. One day, he was sitting at the Pittsburgh airport with a friend who was a young member of the Mellon family. They were in his friend's private jet, a luxurious twenty-seater. Ram Dass was suitably impressed with the plane, commenting on the richness of the interior and its many amenities. "You are very fortunate to have a plane like this," he said to his friend. "Yeah," his friend replied, "but this jet is not as nice as my uncle's jet." He pointed outside to another plane on the tarmac. "It carries forty people and is much nicer. I could never have a jet like that." There is no end to how we can diminish, trivialize, or tarnish our own story if we compare it enviously to other people. In doing so, we not only fail to see the value and nobility in our own story, but we also fail to take into consideration what's behind the story of the people we envy (a lot of people who seem to have everything are desperately broken in some way). When you assess your story, try to look at it exclusive of the influence of others. This is decidedly not a competition.

WRITE IT DOWN

Now you're ready to write. Take out a piece of paper or fire up the computer and write down the most essential things you can understand about your *story behind the story*. Focus on key themes, the things you can appreciate about your life as an epic journey in self-discovery. You won't have to do a lot of writing—two pages at most.

Start, if possible, by identifying your own essential nature. Are you a seeker, teacher, peacemaker, lover, author, scientist, social reformer, nurturer/parent, entrepreneur, statesman, or healer? Perhaps you are a Renaissance man or woman, with more than one "calling" in life. Maybe your goals in life have changed over time. If so, sketch the progression. You want to look at your life as a quest to become what you want to be most.

List the historical triumphs and major roadblocks (persons and events) as they relate to your understanding of who you have been, who you are becoming, and who you want to be. With regard to roadblocks, you'll probably notice some repetitive patterns (life will challenge us repeatedly until we understand the underlying lesson). Revisit your strengths and challenges. Look at your strengths for what they reveal about your nobility—the hero in you—and look at your challenges for what they reveal about your need to change. What are you supposed to understand that you haven't been able to grasp? What are the underlying lessons life is trying to teach you that you have yet to learn?

Go back to the scales in chapter 5 and write a sentence for each that explains why you rated yourself the way you did. For example, if you rated the love in your life as low, ask yourself why and answer it in one sentence (for example, "I responded to my parents' emotional distance by closing my heart and distancing myself from others"). Do this for the scales that measure pain and mobility as well. By now, you have a good idea why you carry pain or lack bodily mobility and functionality. Similarly, write down anything you've learned about metaphorical and symbolic presentation of illness in your body. Do you have severe arthritis because you transferred your emotional inflexibility to your joints? Do you suffer from debilitating lower back pain because you are always in the warrior posture toward life and need a strong back to carry the burden?

Lastly, describe what you want most out of life: financial security, peace, love, courage, acknowledgement, worldly accomplishments, adventure, and so on.

Now sit back for a second and consider what you've just done. You're just like Columbus. You have ventured into uncharted territory, traversed stormy seas, and landed in a remarkable new world. You have discovered your *story behind the story*. Your life will never be the same again.

From this New World, you can address the parts of your story that need to be addressed to improve your health concerns. You can uncover what you need to do to live your story more authentically; you can even change the parts of it you feel need to change. In the chapters that follow, I'll show you how.

Congratulations. This is a momentous time. Give yourself a little while to bask in what you've accomplished and to revel in your discoveries.

Then we'll get started on the road to miraculous health.

PART THREE

TREATMENT

CHAPTER 7

GETTING YOURSELF A LITTLE BETTER RIGHT AWAY

N ow that you've built your skills and learned the keys to self-analysis, it's time for you to heal. In this section, you'll learn a new set of tools—built on the basics you've already learned—that you can utilize to overcome any ailment. After you've experimented with the use of these tools, I will help you customize a treatment plan that works best for your *story behind the story*.

We're going to kick-start the treatment process by taking you through a hypnotic exercise that will help you feel better immediately. We will use hypnosis to cut your stress considerably. I call the exercise the Stressbuster. The process is somewhat similar to the quick-hit exercises we did in the preludes to the early chapters, but exponentially more powerful. If you use the Stressbuster, you will quickly bring ease into your life, feel noticeably better right away, and put yourself on course for recovery. It's easy and a great way to gear up for the treatment methods that follow.

ALL STRESSED OUT

Stress is probably the most serious healthcare problem facing our society. We talk a lot about stress in our culture but we don't do enough to combat it, and most people don't actually have a clear understanding of what it is.

Stress arises when there is an unacceptable disparity between your expectations and your actual experiences. There is such a thing as good stress—the challenges posed in our lives have the potential to enhance our physical and mental functioning. However, chronic and excessive stress eventually causes significant harm to mind and body, and you must deal with it effectively.

Stress is endemic to our society, partly because of the pace we keep and partly because of the endless opportunities at our disposal. These opportunities create very high expectations. Interestingly, in indigent rural societies where opportunity is nonexistent, people live without many necessities. Yet, they also live with little stress because they have no expectations that life should or could be different. A person living in a fashion consistent with his or her own personally accepted expectations has no stress, even if living conditions are adverse.

Stress has both mental and physical components. The mental components include things like anger or rage, fear or terror, fragmented or distorted thinking, impatience, erratic emotional states, memory loss, anxiety, and depression. On the physical side, stress activates the sympathetic leg of the nervous system and the release of stress hormones that amp-up production of adrenaline and divert blood flow to the large muscles. The body needs this power because it "thinks" it has to run away from or fight something. This is the so-called "fight or flight" response. When you are in this response mode, blood flows more to the heart and large muscles and correspondingly less to the digestive system and other vital organs that are not immediately necessary for a fight or flight. We all recognize the immediate effects: dry mouth, motor agitation, sweating, heart palpitations, increased blood pressure, enlarged pupils, sleeplessness, and mental anxiety.

The problem is that our lifestyle is chock full of stressors that keep the fight or flight response constantly active. Constant stress leads to poor digestion, autoimmune problems, glandular disease, poor healing, and poor functioning of critical organs.

The effects of stress are cumulative and insidious. The body and mind have a way of acclimating to chronic stress—until the system can't take it any more and crashes with a mental breakdown, bodily dysfunction, or serious illness. Stress begins in childhood and mounts on us gradually, so gradually that you don't notice the buildup. It's like the old parable about the frog and the pot of water. According to the parable, if you drop a frog in boiling water, it'll jump out immediately. However, if you put a frog in a pot of cool water and then slowly heat the water to boiling, the frog will stay in the pot and cook to death. The same is true with you and stress. If the amount of stress you've accumulated in your life were to hit you all at once, it would be overwhelming, forcing you to deal with it. However, since it comes to you gradually, you don't feel yourself "boiling." This is especially problematic if you already carry illness in your body; you simply cannot afford to carry stress as well.

Stress arises from numerous sources. Heavy responsibilities top the list: unpaid bills, a chronically ill child or spouse, a series of important project deadlines at work when there are too few human resources available, and so on. Difficult relationships are also a culprit—few things in life will stress us more than dealing with an abusive parent or sibling, an unfaithful or deceitful spouse, or an enraged boss.

All major life events—such as a move, a death in the family, or a divorce—are stressful. Even positive events like a wedding or a new baby cause stress. Catastrophic events like car accidents, terrorist bombings, or natural disasters are intensely stressful and debilitating and have severely negative consequences for individuals, families, and entire segments of society.

Our environment also creates stress—too much harsh sound, rush hour traffic, long lines. Societal expectations end up becoming our own, and so we stress as we strive to earn a decent salary, live in a good neighborhood, wear attractive clothes, have perfect hair, own the right car, and be actively involved in the affairs of school, church, and community.

Advanced age and chronic illness are stressful for obvious reasons. As the body fails to rise to the challenges of day-to-day living, the gap between one's experience and one's expectations widens. Chronic pain in and of itself is a major cause of stress. Acute pain of the type experienced during childbirth, injury, or surgery also triggers the human stress response. Stress can also result from poor nutrition, too little sleep, too little exercise, and even by imagined experiences, such as frightening dreams or movies. There is almost no end to the things that stress us out.

I do a lot of work with veterans. About two years ago, a fifty-five-year-old veteran of the Vietnam War came to my office seeking help with his symptoms associated with Post Traumatic Stress Disorder (PTSD), a problem that affects a large number of war veterans involving the subconscious and conscious repetition of trauma and a heightened vulnerability to stress of any kind. Decorated for valor in the military, this man embarked on a successful career as vice president of a major electronics firm after the war, fell in love, married, and started a family, but the symptoms of PTSD haunted him throughout. For thirty years after the war, he never slept through the night. He relived difficult battlefield experiences continuously, especially the day his best friend was blown up right beside him. He had never been able to expunge the guilt he felt for not being able to save his friend and other members of his troop. He was anxious and often angry. Anti-anxiety drugs had done little to help. Try as he did to manage his symptoms, his erratic behavior was harmful to those he loved. His marriage and his relationship with his children literally became casualties of the Vietnam War. The pressure on his heart from chronically high levels of stress eventually manifested as a major heart attack that forced him into early retirement. He had to take it easy after this, living on heart medication and suffering from angina and severe weakness whenever he exerted himself.

He was a virtuous and courageous man and I had an oceanic compassion for him. Our work together involved the use of hypnosis to find and release the battlefield experiences that were continually playing out in his subconscious mind. As we did so, we dismantled the chronic stress-response syndrome that had been fueling his emotional and physical ill health. We also used hypnosis to help him move into super-conscious awareness, where he found the peace and joy that had so long eluded him. He began to meditate regularly. He found his *story behind the story* and began to live it out authentically—his quest was to move away from being a warrior into being a lover. His heart improved to the point where he no longer felt pain or weakness. He began sleeping through the night and stopped relying on anti-anxiety meds. His PTSD symptoms went away entirely, and he went on to find a new career and a new love in his life, free from the stress that had plagued him for decades.

How does this story relate to you? Did you experience extreme difficulty as a child, adolescent, or young adult? The battlefield of life snared many of us when we were young. Much of the anxiety and depression we suffer as adults derives from early life trauma that goes unresolved.

Stress has two stages. First comes the stressful experience itself. Let's say your mother died when you were nine and it was very stressful. The second stage involves how you reacted to it. If your father and extended family were lovingly supportive, they would have helped you understand the loss had nothing to do with you and given you a great deal of nurturing. Dad might even have sent you to a psychologist or bereavement counselor to help you work things out while dad remained a rock-solid symbol of love in your life. If all these things were true, you'd probably be able to heal from the stress created by your mother's death, and you'd develop some good emotional intelligence to boot—you would be a pro at dealing with stressful circumstances later in life.

However, what if life were a lot less loving and a little more complicated after your mother died? Perhaps Dad was too wrapped up in his own suffering to pay attention to your needs and left you on your own to figure out what to do. In this vacuum, you may have responded with any number of likely distortions in thought and feeling: "I must've done something wrong for this to happen ... this is my fault ... I'm going to fry in hell for the argument I had with mom before she died ... I deserved this ... Dad's never going to rally ... gotta take care of Dad and my little brother ... I'm screwed." You'd feel swamped by shame, guilt, confusion, powerlessness, and a sense of abandonment, as if life were over. Those patterns would sink deep into your subconscious mind and continue to haunt you through life. Every time life threw you a curveball—like your boss telling you that your work on an important project was awful—you'd respond with shame, guilt, confusion, powerlessness, a sense of abandonment, and the fear that life was over. If you have early life trauma, abuse, or other extremely stressful circumstances under your belt and you haven't fully dealt with them, you might be more similar to the war veteran than you know.

HOW TO DEAL WITH IT

There are many ways to combat stress. The methods offered in this book have the power to free you from it completely and permanently—regardless of how stressful your life is and how much stress you might be carrying from early in your life. You can be free of it all. In this chapter though, the goal is to knock down the amount of stress you carry by at least 50 percent using one simple hypnotic exercise. This will be a great start, and I promise we'll take care of the rest later.

To understand how this exercise works, you need to understand how best to minimize stress. Two common responses to stress simply won't work well enough for you. The first of these is trying to "think" your way out of a stressful situation. This can be helpful occasionally, but you can't fix every problem with logic. Let's say your problem persists no matter how you analyze it and respond to it logically. If you keep applying logic to an illogical problem, your thinking becomes distorted. At that point, you become like the man who is lost on the back roads of West Virginia, driving left and right, uphill and down, trying to find your way out of the mountains with no map and a broken compass.

The second response that rarely delivers a result is trying to "tough" your way through a stressful situation using willpower. That approach might help you survive the current crisis, but it'll cause even more stress. If stressful events crop up frequently on your radar screen (as they do for most of us), you can't keep overcoming them with willpower alone. At some point, the accumulated stress will catch up with you. You must slow down long enough to deal with it.

That's where the Stressbuster comes in.

To get free from stress, you have to get out of the conscious mind altogether. You have two options available to you. You can use meditation to access super-conscious mind (as we discussed in chapter 4), or you can use imagination and imagery to access the power of the subconscious mind. Meditation will certainly work, but its true benefits come only after you've logged a number of hours in practice. In this chapter, we're going to use hypnotic-guided imagery to access the power of the subconscious mind to free you from stress measurably and *immediately*.

THE STRESSBUSTER

You will come out of this hypnotic exercise feeling unbelievably de-stressed. In fact, you'll probably wind up saying to yourself, "I had no idea I was that stressed to begin with." That's how much better you'll feel afterward.

Download Induction Gamma-I from www.miracuoushealthbook.com. Turn off the phone, dim the lights, set aside as many distractions as you can, get comfortable, and play the download. It will guide you into a hypnotic state that will allow you to melt your stress away.

When you come out of the hypnotic Stressbuster, notice your physical condition. You should feel significantly better. Most people report a 50 percent decrease in pain or a proportionate improvement in the ability to function. Perhaps you can lift your arm higher than you could before, breathe more freely, or climb the stairs without fatigue. If you keep doing this hypnotic exercise, its healing power will gain in potency.

FOLLOWING THE PROGRAM AND GETTING BETTER EVERY DAY

You've already begun to use meditation. If you have been meditating three times per week, you've probably noticed some level of improvement in your physical condition. Now add the Stressbuster to your weekly regimen. You will find the treatment effect to be dramatic. Continue to meditate (or use hypnotically guided meditation if you prefer) three to four times per week and use the Stressbuster on the days in between. Do this for about a week and watch what happens to you. Watch your stress drop and your health improve dramatically. See how happy and joyful you become.

You should also feel yourself charged with positive thinking. You'll find that these methods offer tremendous levels of inspiration because they present you with the promise of what is available to you if you keep going. Consider, as you feel better every day, that the level of improvement you're experiencing is only the tip of the iceberg. You haven't even begun to use the advanced methods you will learn in the coming pages—methods that will take you to miraculous levels of healing.

Your physical ailments may have left you discouraged, stressed, and worried about your condition. You wouldn't be human if you didn't have at least a little concern about your health. However, given what you now know about the power of the mind, you realize that all this worry has been working against you and making it harder for you to recover. With the exercises in this chapter and the genuine improvement you feel, you'll gain momentum and get it going in the right direction. At this point, you should be telling yourself that you *are* getting better. You're worth it; you deserve to be healthy and happy. You know you have the power to accomplish your goals.

And the best is yet to come.

CHAPTER 8

HYPNOTIC PRE-TALK

P eople will go deeply into hypnosis and be able to enjoy its benefits when they know what to expect and how it works. I give this pre-talk to all of my clients as just such an introduction. Read these pages even if you think you know enough about hypnosis already. A good hypnotic pre-talk is *absolutely* essential for success.

I'm going to present this information at two levels—conscious mind and subconscious mind. At a conscious level, you're going to learn a few fascinating things about how the mind works and gain knowledge that will have immediate, positive effects on how you feel. Most of the pre-talk however, "talks" to the subconscious mind to eliminate doubt and other mental blocks that keep a person from going into deep hypnosis and getting the most out of it. In the pages that follow, you'll find me restating a message in different ways and telling a story or using metaphors to bring home a point I've already made. Why? The subconscious mind responds to repetition and "listens" to stories and metaphors. Again, stick with me here. I'm not doing this to show you how much I know; I'm doing it because it will help you. I waited this long to bring this to you because I wanted you to be able to revel in the wonders of the quick-hit methods we did in the preludes to the earlier chapters as rapidly as possible. Now that we're about to dive into the deep water, though, I want you to be fully prepared.

In this chapter, I'm going to dispel the myths about hypnosis and share a few points about the historical evolution of this important clinical tool.

After that, I will describe what hypnosis feels like and say a little bit about the stages of hypnosis. I'll describe the process and tell you how to steer yourself into deep hypnosis so you can enjoy its benefits. After this, you'll be ready to roll.

MYTHS ABOUT HYPNOSIS

You will go deep into hypnosis when you know what it actually is rather than what people think it is. There are several myths about hypnosis in our culture. They result from two sources: misunderstandings regarding outdated hypnotic methods and the daring theater of stage hypnosis.

For at least the last century, people trained in hypnosis were trained in mind control methods, or what's called "authoritarian hypnosis." Hypnotists trained in authoritarian methods were essentially taught to trick a subject (person being hypnotized) into thinking the hypnotist had control of his mind. At that point, the subject relinquished control of his mind because he thought the hypnotist already had it. At the end of the session, the hypnotist would give the subject a post-hypnotic suggestion for amnesia, then bring him out of hypnosis, at which point the subject would say, "Doc where was I?"

Authoritarian hypnosis has *long* been out of use in clinical settings in the United States. Less than 10 percent of the hypnosis done in a therapist's office today uses authoritarian methods. Yet, most of the myths surrounding hypnosis derive from this approach, in part because it survives in the form of stage hypnosis, an entertainment medium. As I mentioned in chapter 3, there's a huge difference between stage hypnotism and therapeutic hypnosis, which is what we're going to be doing.

Authoritarian (mind control) methods aren't effective for everyone. An excellent hypnotist will be able to hypnotize less than 70 percent of people using these methods. They simply don't work on people who, like me, aren't comfortable giving up control. I have a strong mind and am not comfortable giving up control of my pinky finger. If that sounds like you, an authoritarian method wouldn't work on you. One reason the stage shows work is that stage hypnotists pre-screen participants for their degree of "suggestibility." Highly suggestible people tend to respond well to authoritarian methods. Out of those who *can* become hypnotized using these methods, only about a quarter will go into deep hypnosis. That ratio is too small to be useful in the work we're doing together. If you want to get the benefits of hypnosis, you need to be able to go deep.

There are three myths that derive from the popular use of authoritarian methods of hypnosis:

- When hypnotized, you are not in control, but the hypnotist is.
- You are unaware of what is going on around you while you are under hypnosis.
- You will not remember what happened when you were under.

These myths are artifacts of the authoritarian method. If you don't use that means of transport, you don't get those results. We are not using authoritarian methods, so you will remain in complete control.

We are using state-of-the-art clinical methods. Using these methods, you'll be in control the whole time, fully aware of what's happening, and will remember everything; you're running the show.

From about 1978 to 1985, the field of clinical hypnosis shifted away from the use of authoritarian methods to the use of "permissive methods." In 1978, the baby boom generation came into power—the first of the anti-authoritarian generations to have followed the shift in clinical methods. We were anti-government, anti-war, and anti-discrimination. And in clinical circles, we were anti-mind control. And we were right to feel that way. It's just not a very good idea to try to take control of someone else's mind. Free will is what drives enlightenment.

At the end of the 1970s, the entire field shifted to permissive methods. Progressive Relaxation (PR) methods that rely heavily on the use of guided imagery are the most common permissive approach used in hypnosis. I used PR in chapter 7 (a warm relaxing feeling washes over you as you lay on a tropical beach listening to the waves rushing onto the shore). Nearly 80 percent of the hypnotic inductions done in a therapist's office today use PR methods. Why? They're easy, permissive (they keep the client in control), and relaxing, so people tend to like them. About 90 percent of people go into hypnosis using permissive methods. The reason this percentage is higher than the percentage that go into hypnosis using authoritarian methods is because it includes the people who are uncomfortable giving up control. The 10 percent that still don't go into hypnosis with permissive methods are people who have trouble relaxing.

By the late 1980s, the field of clinical hypnosis began to shift into a third phase of evolution based on the latest brain research. The result: the state-of-the-art clinical hypnosis used today by advanced practitioners in clinical settings. We will be doing this type of hypnosis. We'll be using permissive methods, where you're in control, along with state-of-the-art techniques for deepening your trance state. Using this approach, close to 100 percent of people go into deep hypnosis rapidly without going to sleep, and with these methods, you can relax your way in or control your way in, whatever you prefer.

Ninety percent of people will get a nice, relaxed feeling from the methods that we'll be using. Often, when I take someone into hypnosis and bring them out, they go on and on about what a wonderfully relaxed feeling they have, but technically "feeling relaxed" is a byproduct of hypnosis and not the purpose of hypnosis itself. Some people don't get fully relaxed, especially if they go into the process with a lot of mental or bodily stress. If you're one of these people, you'll still go into deep hypnosis, and once you accomplish what you need to do under hypnosis, your stress (and even the pain in your body) will go away.

That leads me to two other myths about hypnosis: that hypnosis and relaxation are one and the same and that you have to be relaxed in order to go deeply into hypnosis. Baloney. If hypnosis and relaxation were the same, we wouldn't bother with hypnosis; we'd send people to the beach and tell them to get a massage or soak in a Jacuzzi. This is patently absurd, yet you'll hear it from practitioners who I believe aren't sufficiently trained. You have to be relaxed in order to be hypnotized only if you're using relaxation-based methods like PR. With the methods we'll be using, you'll go deep regardless.

Now let's look at two other concerns that might keep a person from going into very deep hypnosis. First, people often wonder if they're capable of being hypnotized. Without even knowing you, I can tell you that the answer is yes. Everyone can be hypnotized. Hypnosis is a naturally occurring state of human consciousness. We all go in and out of hypnosis throughout the day (a fact I explore in the next section of this chapter). If you tried hypnosis, it failed because your hypnotherapist wasn't terribly good or you didn't really want to succeed. "I can't be hypnotized" is something I hear often from people just before I hypnotize them deeply for the first time. If you want to try hypnosis and you have a well-trained clinical guide, it'll work for you.

A second common concern arises in people who worry that, once they're hypnotized, they'll be caught in it and won't be able to get back. Impossible—it takes the ongoing voice of the hypnotherapist to keep you under, or else you pop out of hypnosis within a few minutes or fall asleep and wake up feeling refreshed ten minutes later. Of course, there is a very deep level of hypnosis that is so joyful and healing to mind and body that you might not *want* to get out of it. I get people into these states quite often, at which point they usually say, "Don't bring me out now, Rick. This is fabulous. I don't want to come back!" However, you cannot stay under hypnosis without the aid of the hypnotherapist. You cannot be *caught in hypnosis*.

WHAT DOES IT FEEL LIKE?

Some people think that when you're in hypnosis you feel like you're in some weird altered dream state. Nothing could be further from the truth. A person under hypnosis is very focused and aware of what they're concentrating on.

We all move through hypnotic states, at varying levels of depth, every day. There are three basic levels of hypnotic depth: deep, moderate and light.

Everyone goes into deep hypnosis right before falling asleep (the hypnogogic state) and just before waking up (the hypnopompic state). Your mind does not go directly from being awake to being asleep, or vice versa. Instead, you transition from being awake, to deep hypnosis, and then sleep; when asleep, you must go through deep hypnosis in order to wake up. If you couldn't enter into deep hypnosis, you wouldn't be able to fall asleep or wake up. If you sleep every night, you're experiencing deep hypnosis at least twice a day.

We are all familiar with moderate hypnotic states. In chapter 3, I gave the well-known example of highway hypnosis: you pull into the driveway and can't remember the drive home. Anytime you do something on "autopilot" without consciously thinking about it, you are in a moderate state of waking hypnosis—while your conscious mind is completely preoccupied with something, the subconscious mind takes over and gets the job done, and you are barely aware of it. Haven't you ever started a mundane task, such as doing the dishes after Thanksgiving dinner, when your thoughts drift off, and before you know it, the dishes are done and you hardly remember doing them? That's moderate hypnosis.

Light hypnotic states occur very frequently. For example, let's say you're typing on your laptop on an important project at your nearby cybercafé or Starbucks. It's lunchtime, and there's a lot of hubbub in the background—music, patrons bustling around, baristas handling coffee orders—but you are so focused on your work, you hear none of it. The sound just fades away as if it doesn't exist. That's a common light hypnotic state.

So, you're already drifting through hypnotic states naturally throughout the day. These natural hypnotic states are called "waking hypnosis." When delivered by a trained hypnotherapist, it's called "formal hypnosis." However, it's the same darn state of mind, no matter how you enter it.

Therefore, when you go into hypnosis it will not seem like some strange altered state to you. You'll respond by thinking, "Oh, I'm already familiar with that. I didn't call it hypnosis, but now I get it." You're doing it every day, many times a day, and now you're going to learn how to manage your access and apply it in ways that benefit you immensely.

So What the Heck *Is* It?

Now that we've debunked the myths about hypnosis, we'll answer the question "What is it?" I'm going to give you a clinical definition of hypnosis and then explain what it's all about.

Hypnosis is "critical factor bypass through the establishment of acceptable selective thinking." I know; that's a mouthful. Let's put it into plain English.

First, let's go back to our working model of the mind, which has three parts: the conscious, subconscious, and super-conscious minds. The conscious mind, the smallest and weakest part of the mind, is composed of conscious analytical reason. The subconscious mind is many times the size and power of the conscious mind, a storehouse of old memories, symbols, feelings, and deep understandings about who you are and what your purpose in life is. The super-conscious mind is infinite in power, allowing you to influence your own destiny, other people, places, and events, as well as merge with the ocean of energy that sustains the entire universe.

For reasons I explained at length in prior chapters, you need to be able to access the content of the subconscious and super-conscious minds if you want to achieve your goals for self-healing. Hypnosis will let you accomplish this by allowing you to get past the mental barriers that prevent access to the subconscious and super-conscious minds.

Access to the subconscious mind is blocked by a "gatekeeper," a psychological wall that stops what is in the subconscious mind from going into conscious mind, and vice versa. In the course of day-to-day affairs, you *want* to have the gatekeeper in place. Otherwise, every memory, every old song you ever heard, would be cropping up in the back of your mind twenty-four hours a day, seven days a week. You would be so distracted you wouldn't be able to concentrate. As it is, the gatekeeper is permeable and memories slip through. Remember in the old days when DJs used to play the same songs repeatedly? The subconscious mind responds to repetition. There was one song called "Little Star" ("There you are, little star"). I must've heard it a hundred times on the radio. After that, it was always pushing past my gatekeeper. To this day, I will be walking along or driving and out of nowhere, "There you are, little star" comes blowing into my mind. What an intrusion—I hated that song! You want your gatekeeper to work. You want to be able to block this kind of thing out.

The gatekeeper also makes decisions about what will be allowed to go back and forth between the conscious and subconscious minds. Often, we're working on an issue in the subconscious mind and totally unaware of it. The issue may show up in a dream, but dreams are often unintelligible. How often have you awakened from a dream and thought, "My God, that didn't make any sense at all"? After you start to make progress on this issue, though the gatekeeper says, "All right, it's OK to know this at a conscious level," and that's when you become aware of the issue. So, the gatekeeper is constantly making critical judgments about what's allowed to go back and forth.

The technical clinical name of this gatekeeper is the "critical factor." If you're going to go from your conscious mind to your subconscious mind, which is what happens in hypnosis, you've got to bypass that gatekeeper. In other words, you must achieve "critical factor bypass" (the first part of our clinical definition).

What achieves that bypass? According to the definition above, it's "the establishment of acceptable selective thinking." This is just a technical way of saying we achieve gatekeeper bypass by using hypnotic suggestions that fit your values. If the hypnotic method does not use suggestions that fit your values, you will not go into hypnosis. The types of suggestions we will be using here are simple and basic, designed to fit everyone's values.

In the end, there is just one thing you have to do to go into deep hypnosis: bypass the gatekeeper (using suggestions that fit your values). If you do this, you will quite naturally access the subconscious mind, go deep into hypnosis, and get the job done, no matter what your goal is. Hypnosis is simply a way of directing your thought process to bypass the gatekeeper and get into the subconscious mind. Once there, you can relieve yourself of the things that hold you back and tap into the power and vision of the subconscious mind. It's that simple, and you will find yourself making meaningful progress with it quickly.

Access to the super-conscious mind is blocked by a second gatekeeper (or critical factor) between the subconscious and super-conscious minds. This gatekeeper controls how much super-conscious awareness is moving into the subconscious mind—and from there into conscious mind.

You may ask why it would be necessary for this gatekeeper to be in place. Wouldn't everyone want this gatekeeper to be open given what the super-conscious mind has to offer? As wondrous as that sounds, the untrained mind could not stand the billion megawatts of power that would pipe through a fully open door to super-consciousness. We get what we can handle. As you go deeper and deeper into the process you're learning in this book, you'll gain greater and greater access to it, because your mind and body will become incredibly strong.

Rest assured, the gatekeeper to super-consciousness is permeable. If this gatekeeper were not partially open, you could not draw a breath—your heart wouldn't beat. A substantial minority of persons, for example those of great faith and those who meditate regularly, have a measurable degree of super-conscious awareness—for them, the gatekeeper is highly permeable. Everyone's gatekeeper allows super-consciousness to "peep" through now and then, as evidenced by surveys showing that more than two-thirds of us have had a major life-changing psychic or religious experience.

The exercises in this book, the meditative ones in particular, are designed to strengthen and tune the mind so it can accommodate super-conscious power and awareness. Deep hypnotic states can be used to facilitate super-conscious access by calming, focusing, and strengthening your awareness, at which point the gatekeeper relaxes and slides out of the way because it is no longer necessary; you can then perceive the levels of intuitive thought that you need to experience universal wisdom and power.

THE PROCESS

Most hypnotic experiences have three parts: an induction, a hypnotic experience, and an emergence. The first part is an induction, a formalized group of words, phrases, and imagery that move your attention away from the outside world and toward a relaxed and focused inner awareness. This process naturally moves you past both gatekeepers. The inductions I use involve a basic focusing and relaxing procedure, often a ten-to-one count-down using a variety of voice modulations and prompts and a few simple PR methods to help relax body and mind.

The second stage of hypnosis is the hypnotic experience itself. I will guide you to a memory, an issue, or another location in your mind or body using imagery, direct suggestion, or a combination of these methods. Once you've arrived at your destination, you will naturally experience the wisdom, power, and perception of the subconscious (or super-conscious) mind. You will merge right in. Some people move back and forth between subconscious and super-conscious awareness, depending on the nature of their inquiry. For example, if you are trying to reverse an old habit of thought that is keeping you ill, you will be exploring the subconscious mind almost exclusively. However, if your health problem has to do with meaning-of-life issues, you may move back and forth between the subconscious and super-conscious minds, as both will have insight to offer.

After you complete your experience, I will emerge you from the hypnotic state. Emerging is a simple process that involves a one-to-five count and direct suggestions that guide you back to a normal waking state of consciousness. At that point, you will remember everything about your experience.

Once you've done this process a few times, it becomes easy. You'll just float right in.

HOW TO STEER YOURSELF IN

I'm your guide in this process and I am very good at what I do, but you are in the driver's seat. You are the one in control, and you must do a few things to get the most out of hypnosis.

First, assume the right attitude: "I like this; I'm doing it." We have precisely this attitude toward anything we naturally desire and enjoy. I feel this way about hiking, basketball, physics, and travel. Think of anything you really enjoy doing and consider your attitude about it, whether it is cooking, sports, dance, swimming, regular massages—anything you naturally take to and want to do without doubt or hesitation. That is a natural hypnotic state for anyone. "I like it; I'm doing it." When you're feeling that way, you've got your entire mind working for you.

Deep hypnosis requires bypass of the gatekeeper(s); bypass requires the attitude, "I like it; I'm doing it." There are four different types of attitudes that have been studied for their ability or inability to bypass the gatekeeper:

- Conscious attitude 1: "I like it, I'm doing it." If you take that attitude, you'll succeed every time.
- Conscious attitude 2: "I disagree with it." This will obviously kick you right out of hypnosis.
- Conscious attitude 3: "I'm neutral about it." This won't work either. This is the type of attitude you take when you're overweight and you say to yourself, "Oh gee, I guess maybe that broccoli and cauliflower diet could work for me."
- Conscious attitude 4: This is the one you have to watch out for. The attitude is, "I like it; I'm gonna try it," or, "I like it; I hope it's gonna work." Such an attitude will result in sure failure every time because "trying" and "hoping" are not enough. Trying and hoping introduce a little

bit of doubt or fear to the mind. Think about your success with the mind-body methods instead of failure.

The thing about the subconscious mind is that it can't differentiate between what's actually going on and what is being heard or seen. The subconscious mind doesn't have good contact with the external world. It relies on conscious mind to interpret and is "suggestible" to conscious input. An applicable and well-researched example is the professional basketball player who wants to improve his shooting percentage. In comparative studies, pro players were exposed to three different training regimens: practice on the court shooting baskets, practice accompanied by watching a video of successful shots, and watching video of successful shots alone. The athletes who only watched the video improved their shooting percentages the most because the other two training methods (which quite naturally involved some missed shots) introduced an element of failure to the subconscious mind.

So, the subconscious mind will accept what you say, even if you're feeling a little doubt or fear. If you affirm, "I like this; I'm doing it" with any degree of confidence whatsoever, you will convince the subconscious mind to accept it.

The second thing you need to do to go in deep and get the most out of hypnosis is to use imagination, not willpower. Willpower won't work—that's a tool of the conscious mind. Willpower is great if it's 11:30 P.M. and you're looking at a sink full of dirty dishes; it will help you get the dishes done. However, if you rely on willpower under hypnosis, you will sabotage yourself because it will keep you locked in the conscious mind. Whatever suggestion is given during a hypnotic induction, do not try to "will" it into effect. Just imagine it coming into being. Einstein said, "Imagination, not reason, is the key to knowledge." He knew what he was talking about. If I ask you to relax during a hypnotic induction and you try to will it into being, you will "freeze up." Just imagine that you're relaxed, ease into it, and it will happen.

A third key to successful hypnosis is to just let the experience unfold without second-guessing or over-analyzing the process while you're in it. There'll be plenty of time for that later. You will find that your experience under hypnosis is very real and authentic, if you allow it. You may move into an active stance or a passive stance. In the active stance, you'll be thinking up and answering questions. In the passive stance, you'll feel more like you are watching a movie or "receiving" thought or impressions. Any combination of these experiences is valid.

A lot of people expect to experience powerful imagery—Panavision with surround sound—and when they don't get that, they get frustrated and shut down the experience. You may get Panavision and you may not. Highly rational people tend to experience hypnotic insight, even memory, more as thoughts or ideas. Some people get symbolic expressions only. With a little practice, your means of perception under hypnosis will evolve, and you'll be able to experiment with many different states of awareness.

A last key to your success concerns how to deal with a situation where my idea of "acceptable thinking" and yours do not agree. In the hypnotic downloads that accompany this book I have attempted to utilize language that is universally acceptable to all people. However, if at any time I say something that rubs you the wrong way during the hypnotic process, then ignore it and reformulate it with something that will fit your values. Create and accept your own re-interpretation right in the moment. You are fully present in the process. You know what's going on while you're doing hypnosis, and you will help yourself by adapting in this way.

This is how you steer yourself:

- Have the right attitude.
- Use imagination rather than willpower.
- Let the experience unfold.
- Reformulate any suggestions that might not fit your values.

With a little practice, this will become second nature to you, and you will easily merge into deep hypnotic experience.

I hope the methods you've already learned have brought you great levels of improved health, peace and, wellbeing. Even so, you've only seen the warm-up act. You're now ready to experience true "powerhouse" methods of self-healing.

Let's get to the main attraction.

CHAPTER 9

COMBINING DIRECT SUGGESTION
AND HEALING IMAGERY
UNDER HYPNOSIS

N ow that you have a good understanding of hypnosis and some experience with this powerful clinical tool, you can begin to use hypnosis for
specific healing purposes. In this chapter, I will introduce you to hypnotic
methods that combine direct suggestion and healing imagery to accomplish
three specific goals:

- Identifying and removing illness from the body
- Relieving pain
- Losing weight

Each of these methods has considerable power. Which ones you use and
how often you use them will depend on your individual needs and preferences. If you experiment with these methods, you will know whether or not
they are right for you and be able to customize their use to suit your needs.

Before starting, review your self-assessments from chapters 5 and 6,
especially the self-rating scales in chapter 5. These constitute your general
wellness baseline, and as you move forward to utilize the tools in the

remainder of the book, you'll want to keep track of your progress against this baseline. Bring in any other information you have about your health at this point, as well. For instance, if you are a diabetic, you know your blood sugar level; if you have heart problems, you know your resting blood pressure and cholesterol levels; if you have glaucoma, you have the results of your last eye exam, and so on. Any hard medical data you have at your disposal—a recent X-ray, MRI, PET scan, CAT scan, lab work, or physician's report, for example—should be part of your baseline. Having this baseline allows you to measure your progress as you go and will give you a greater say in your own healthcare.

THE TECHNIQUES IN THIS CHAPTER

The methods in this chapter rely on a combination of two commonly used hypnotic techniques: direct suggestion and guided healing imagery. Direct suggestion, as the name implies, involves the use of positive suggestions to the mind under hypnosis. As I mentioned in chapter 8, we will only use suggestions that fit your values. The direct suggestions we'll be using are simple, clinically appropriate, and universally acceptable, such as, "There's a great feeling of ease, comfort, and strength growing inside of you." Suggestions like this one simply equate with positive thinking. When you use positive thinking under hypnosis, the effect is *exponentially* greater than when you use it in a waking conscious state.

Virtually everyone is aware of the power of positive thinking and the notion that if you believe good things are going to happen to you, they will. There is a great deal of truth to this notion, and as we have discussed elsewhere, it is a wise move to maintain a positive attitude toward health and healing. However, chances are that you are *not* going to get yourself better simply by thinking good thoughts about your health. If that were all that was necessary, you would have healed yourself already.

Remember, most people "think" only at a conscious level, and conscious mind is the smallest part of the mind. The subconscious mind is nearly three times as large and powerful, and you're actively "thinking" there, too. If the subconscious mind is stubbornly holding onto the idea of disease in the body, no amount of positive thinking at a conscious level is going to turn the tide.

Understanding this can help you avoid needless suffering. Just last year a forty-two-year-old mother of two young girls came to see me. She was suffering from lymphoma and had just finished a yearlong course of very intensive chemotherapy that had had *no* positive clinical effect, according to her doctor. "I don't understand it," she said. "I have the best medical care, the best nutrition, and I've been listening to positive affirmation tapes and feeling very optimistic about my health—I was certain I was going to get better." Under hypnosis, this woman discovered that her subconscious mind had a strongly different view. Her mother had died from cancer when she was little, and she was still holding on to the idea that she was somehow responsible for her mother's death. Not only that, but her marriage of twelve years to a man who suffered from frequent bouts of rage had been more painful and disappointing than she was willing to acknowledge at a conscious level. Her subconscious mind had "given up" under the weight of so much emotional pain. It was actively working against her recovery and her "conscious optimism" to such an extent that the effects of her excellent medical treatment had been sabotaged.

Prevent negative subconscious thinking from sabotaging you. You have to get *both* the conscious mind and the subconscious mind to "think positively" if you want to get better. One highly efficient way to do this is through direct suggestion under hypnosis. Under hypnosis, the door to the subconscious mind is open, and the subconscious mind is likely to agree to and adopt acceptable positive suggestions for healing.

The other technique we'll be using—guided healing imagery—has power for reasons that should now be obvious to you. As I mentioned in chapter 3, the "native language" of the subconscious mind is imagery, metaphor, and feeling. Symbolic imagery, therefore, provides a direct link to the subconscious mind and can be utilized under hypnosis as a means to activate the latent storehouse of mental power you possess there.

Highly cognitive people who learn best through logic will tend to respond well to direct suggestion. Sensory-oriented individuals who have a strong awareness of imagery (artists, designers, and so on) tend to learn best through visual and other sensory stimuli and will respond well to the use of guided healing imagery. The combination of these two techniques under hypnosis offers a "way in" for both types of learners.

Under hypnosis, even highly cognitive types will be able use imagery to access the power in the subconscious. Take me, for example. I am not very sensory-oriented. I'm so cognitive, in fact, that I can't figure out how to best arrange the furniture in my living room. Under hypnosis, I don't experience imagery with Panavision, surround sound, or other types of sensory experience. If you are like me, you can "think" your way through guided imagery under hypnosis. Just "think it" into being. It works for me; it'll work for you.

Sensory-oriented creative types will find it easy to adopt positive direct suggestions under hypnosis accompanied by imagery. If this is your case, you'll find that the direct suggestions just *slide* into the subconscious mind while it is being entertained by sensory experience brought on via healing imagery.

The bottom line: combining direct suggestion and guided healing imagery under hypnosis will allow the vast majority of people to achieve dramatic results.

REMOVING ILLNESS FROM THE BODY

This hypnotic method will allow your mind to use its power to remove illness from your body. Too many people who suffer from chronic or catastrophic illness have come to see themselves as powerless against their ailments. This method counteracts that. It'll be good for your self-esteem, good for your sense of personal empowerment, and it'll work by getting your subconscious and super-conscious minds actively working with you in the fight against the disease and mental disharmony you carry.

Here's a huge point for you to understand at this stage in your treatment: the number one rule in healing is that you heal yourself through love. Remember that. As we've discussed, the illness in your body has a mental root related to your *story behind the story*. You want to counteract the distorted thinking that hinders you without setting up a situation where you feel as though you're attacking yourself. Look at what you're now embarking on in a balanced way: there is a noble, powerful, unique "you" that exists quite apart from the distortions in thought and feeling that have contributed to your illness. This "you" is worthy of your constant love, respect, and admiration. Remember to give yourself that love. It is *so* important to your healing.

As far as the distortion is concerned, however, you don't need to give that any love at all. This method will allow you to confront the illness in your body in a strong way. It'll free you from a sense of powerlessness ("Why is this happening to me?") and move you into a sense of potency and self-control ("I can do something about it").

Get yourself ready for this exercise. Kick back and relax for a moment. Then, imagine a metaphor or symbol you can associate with your ailment. Next, think about how you're going to overcome this ailment using the same symbolism and write your concept down on a piece of paper. You will be using this imaginative approach under hypnosis.

I'll give you a couple of very different examples of what I'm talking about. I once had a patient who was a retired army colonel with major heart problems. As he focused on his heart, he imagined two armies: the good guys in white uniforms (representing his good health) and the bad guys in black uniforms (representing his disease). Under hypnosis, he imagined the good soldiers gaining ground over the territory of his heart and the evil soldiers fleeing in all directions (out of his heart and out of his body). This approach fit the colonel's values, worked well for him, and might work well for you.

On the other hand, something at the other end of the spectrum might be more useful to you. I once treated a musician who had leukemia. He was a gentle, artistic sort. When we used this method, he envisioned wave after wave of pure clean water washing over his head and through his body to his feet. Every wave carried its own musical note, and the progression of waves formed a lilting melody. As each wave landed at his feet, it carried some portion of his cancer with it, washing him clean of the disease.

Find imagery that fits your worldview and preferences. If the imagery you use the first time doesn't fit well, you can change it midcourse while you're under hypnosis or try something different the next time you use the method.

Download Induction Gamma-II from www.miraculoushealthbook.com, burn it onto a CD, and set up the room the way you have for the other hypnotic exercises. This experience will move you through an induction, then take you through a few minutes of direct suggestions designed to empower you for self-healing, and lastly, prompt you to run your healing imagery in your mind for about ten minutes. After that, I will emerge you from the experience.

Be aware that the "imagery" that springs to mind during this process might not be visual at all. It could be an inspiring piece of music, a soothing aroma, a pleasant taste, or even a series of ideas. Strongly cognitive people will experience subconscious wisdom more as ideas or thoughts and less as sensory awareness. If that is your experience, stick with it. It will still be helpful.

Many people take to this method right away. Those of you who are more cognitive might need a little practice with the method before you feel its power. I encourage you to experiment with it because it is very potent and you can get a lot from it. Even the most cognitive people can benefit from the method, and the power of it grows with use.

PAIN RELIEF

If you are in chronic pain, you know it's making you miserable in many ways. You can drop that pain dramatically—even remove it altogether—using hypnosis.

Only sufferers of acute pain that is chronic and long in duration know how bad life can get. I know because I've been there. Nearly thirty years ago, I got a burr under my saddle to get in great physical shape. I decided to work the Royal Canadian Air Force Exercise Program and took to it with zeal. I achieved my goal: I had the strength and endurance of a young soldier in top military condition, but my great achievement was shortly eclipsed by my foolishness. I severely damaged my lumbar spine trying to lift too much weight at the gym, and what a price I paid! For most of the year that followed, I lived at a level of pain that, on a scale of one to ten, was about nine and a half. Narcotic painkillers didn't even touch it, nor did anti-inflammatories or physical therapy. Every moment of every day was an excruciating exercise in survival.

When you sink this low, you tend to cave to woeful skepticism about life. Hypnosis has the power to free you from this type of living hell. If only I had had a good method for hypnotic pain relief available to me in my youth!

There has been extensive research on hypnosis for its many benefits to mind and body and most thoroughly for its ability to create analgesia (pain relief) and anesthesia (total lack of feeling). Hypnosis alleviates the pain associated with cancer, neurological problems, orthopedic disorders, migraines, and other chronic conditions. It will also reduce or eliminate acute pain of the sort experienced during catastrophic injuries, childbirth, or painful medical procedures like surgery.

Hypnotic pain relief has many benefits. As any neurologist will tell you, chronic acute pain inflames nerve endings and otherwise "conditions" the nervous system to be hypersensitive to pain. Hypnotic pain relief allows the nervous system to relax and regain normal functioning. This will help you recover more quickly. If you are a chronic pain sufferer, you spend *a lot* of mental and physical energy on pain management and endurance. Hypnotic pain relief will free you from that drain and liberate your mental and physical energy so you can use it to speed your healing along. Hypnotic pain relief also brings with it renewed optimism and faith and can substantially lift the depression and anxiety that frequently accompany chronic pain. And all these benefits of hypnosis come without the negative side effects of chemical analgesics, anti-inflammatories, and anesthetics.

Before we move on to the method, a very important note of caution is in order. This method is extremely powerful. For reasons I explain below, you can use it to alleviate pain *whether or not* you have dealt with the underlying cause of your pain. Pain exists for a reason; it's a built-in alert system, letting you know that something is wrong. If you are in chronic pain and haven't already done so, you'll want to check with a healthcare professional to make sure you're getting the essential healthcare that's appropriate for your condition.

Use this method for its healthful benefits, not to mask underlying symptoms or as an excuse to avoid appropriate medical care.

This method works by convincing the mind that pain in the body does not exist. Thousands of women who've relied on hypnosis for pain-free childbirth will tell you that they didn't feel anything but pressure. How could that be?

The mind-body connection provides the answer. You can't feel pain if the mind is impervious to it. If there is too little energy in the nervous system, the body cannot communicate the sensation of pain to the central nervous system and brain. No communication, no pain. For example, when I injured my back many years ago, I kept re-injuring it in my sleep because there is very little energy in the nervous system when we're asleep. In sleep, my brain wasn't receiving the "message" that my back was in pain, so I tossed around and hurt myself again.

General anesthesia works the same way. The flow of energy through the central nervous system and brain is so dampened that you feel no pain, even in surgery. At the subatomic level, the mind, brain, and nervous system are one. The mind is capable of dampening or even ceasing the flow of energy in the body. If the mind refuses to acknowledge or receive pain impulses from the nervous system, it is as if those impulses do not exist.

A number of years ago, a man came to see me who had stomach cancer and was undergoing chemotherapy. He lived in extreme chronic pain and was struggling to remain at his job as supervisor of a military supply depot where there were huge demands placed on him for strength, endurance, and agility. When he arrived for his first appointment, he couldn't even walk up a wheelchair ramp. Immediate pain relief was crucial in his case. I taught him the hypnotic method I'm about to teach you. Over a number of weeks, he became free of pain entirely. At work, he returned to his robust former self, walking at different angles, carrying heavy crates, and climbing over stock in the warehouse like a young kid. We, of course, still had to get to his *story behind the story* to discover the root cause of his disease, but in the meantime, he was free to enjoy a more robust quality of life and better pursue his goals for improved health because the excruciating pain was gone.

Why should you continue to be in pain? We are going to drop your pain dramatically right now with the use of this hypnotic exercise. Download Induction Gamma-III from www.miraculoushealthbook.com, burn it onto a CD, and set up the space and time you need for a hypnotic session. This process will start with an induction and then take you through a series of direct suggestions and guided imagery designed to create full-body analgesia (complete relief from pain). If you are in chronic pain, you'll want to use this method every day for a while until you get complete relief. Then use it *pro re nata* (PRN), which in Latin means "as medically necessary" or "at the patient's prerogative."

WEIGHT LOSS

Nearly two-thirds of Americans are obese or overweight. Excess weight is a culprit in the onset and severity of many health problems: hypertension, high cholesterol, Type-2 diabetes, coronary heart disease, stroke, gallbladder disease, osteoarthritis, respiratory problems, and some cancers (endometrial, breast, and colon). Excessive weight also complicates symptoms associated with neurological and orthopedic problems. If your health is poor and you want to recover, you cannot carry excess weight. For all these reasons, I close this chapter with a hypnotic weight loss method.

Hypnosis is clinically proven to result in weight loss. The hypnotic method I offer here will help you shed up to twenty-five pounds. Use it only if you need to lose weight to improve your health and wellbeing. Obviously, do not employ it in order to go below the "healthy weight" your doctor recommends for your height, frame, age, and gender. This method works best in concert with a healthy, balanced lifestyle that includes a low-fat diet and exercise. It will facilitate your weight loss goals but will not replace common sense or compensate for self-destructive behaviors like binge eating.

In this case, we will use direct suggestion combined with guided healing imagery to "convince" your subconscious mind to engage only in healthy behaviors that support your weight loss objectives. There are many good diet and exercise plans available. If you want to lose weight and have been trying good methods yet failed, you should do two things. First, see your doctor to rule out endocrine or other problems that make it difficult to lose weight. Treating a physical problem might help you achieve weight loss. Second, try this hypnotic weight loss exercise.

For any important objective you want to pursue in life, you need to get the power of the subconscious mind working for you. Let's face it: weight loss is hard (especially as you get older). You need all the power you can muster to achieve your weight loss goals. If your subconscious mind is working against you, it will be very difficult, if not impossible, for you to succeed.

There are many reasons why the subconscious mind might sabotage your attempts to lose weight. A common source of subconscious sabotage is abuse or neglect early in life. If unresolved, sadness, fear, anger, guilt, or shame that arises in childhood can perpetuate a subconscious hunger for nurture and love that we satisfy with food. Subconscious emotional pain of this type also fuels poor self-esteem and a sense of powerlessness, which can create a subconscious impulse to gain weight as a means to "save" one's self from a fruitless struggle for happiness.

Those who hold subconscious fear of relationships might overeat in order to create a barrier to human interaction. Alternatively, some people feel weak and small in life, and weight gain actually makes them feel larger and more powerful. Others of us are so stressed at a subconscious level, we eat for emotional reasons. And for some of us, an upbringing characterized by too much junk food and too little exercise ends up establishing a repetition compulsion in the subconscious mind that insists on maintaining the unhealthy pattern, no matter what. These are just a few of the myriad ways in which your subconscious might be working against you in your efforts to lose weight.

The subconscious mind's hold on the body can have some astounding consequences. Many years ago, a lovely woman in her mid-forties came to me with an interesting problem. She was about fifty pounds overweight and wanted to do something about this. Under her doctor's supervision, she had been diligently following a stringent weight-loss plan of only 1,200 calories a day for three months. She had not cheated on her diet and engaged regularly in moderate exercise, but she actually put on three pounds. Her doctor was stupefied. Her situation defied logic, but her unusual circumstances also persuaded her that her weight problem had a mental component, which made her open to the idea of trying hypnosis to find an answer.

Under hypnosis, she revealed that her father had been very emotionally distant while she was growing up. She became a people pleaser in an effort to gain his love and attention. From there, she'd been through a string of failed relationships with men, and these led her to conclude that love relationships just weren't ever going to work for her. Her subconscious mind fixed on the distortion "If I am attractive, men will like me, I'll get involved, and I'll just keep getting hurt." This distortion was keeping her overweight and unattractive, despite her ultra-low calorie intake.

When she found this distortion, she freed herself from it by realizing that she could find healthy love with a man. Hypnotic work to release her early life distortion combined with the method I am about to show you (hypnotic direct suggestion and guided imagery for weight loss) allowed this woman to take control of her life, achieve her ideal weight, and move forward into a better future.

To use the hypnotic weight loss method, download Induction Gamma-IV from www.miraculoushealthbook.com, burn it onto a CD, and set up your room the way you have for the other hypnotic exercises. This experience will move you through an induction, then take you through several minutes of direct suggestions designed to strengthen your self-concept, build respect for your body, increase your control over your future, and adhere to healthy eating habits. After that, I will emerge you from the experience.

Try doing this exercise every day until you begin to see results (reduced hunger, better eating habits, increased vitality, better self-esteem, and weight loss). If excessive weight gain has been a problem for you, you will want to include this method as part of the customized treatment approach that I will help you develop in subsequent chapters.

USE OF THESE METHODS

Rely on one or more of these three methods to the degree that they fit your objectives and deliver the desired healing effect. Virtually everyone will benefit from Induction Gamma-II for removing illness from the body. Experiment with this, customize it to suit your learning style, and incorporate it in your treatment plan if it feels right for you. If chronic pain is an issue for you, adopt Induction Gamma-III for pain relief as part of your treatment plan now. Use it every day until you get substantial relief from pain, then every other day, and then less often on an as-needed basis. If excessive weight is an issue for you, adopt Induction Gamma-IV as part of your treatment regimen now and use it every day until you get results.

Remember, you're both the therapist and the patient here. Trust your own judgment. If one method feels great while another seems uncomfortable or ineffective, go with the one that feels best and stick with it.

As you go through the methods in this book, remember that the goal is to pull together a treatment plan designed to fit your personal needs—a plan that will lead you to miraculous health. We are all different, and therefore, each of us will approach treatment differently. My job is to introduce you to a variety of highly effective methods and let you try them on for size. I'll provide you with insight regarding the methods that might work best for you, but as I tell all of my clients, the choice of how to use them is ultimately yours.

As you move through the chapters that follow, I will continue to introduce you to new methods. The power of any method increases with use over time, and the power you can unleash in yourself by combining methods will, quite frankly, knock your socks off.

CHAPTER 10

HYPNOTIC REGRESSION

M any particularly intransigent physical injuries or illnesses are fueled by mental dis-ease caused by difficult events that occurred in your past. Everyone reading this book has had to endure one or more significant challenges in life, and some of you have had more than your fair share. In this chapter, I provide you with a hypnotic method that allows you to go back in time to revisit the challenges of the past, mine them for what they have to say about your *story behind the story*, and free yourself from the distortions that resulted from a painful experience early in life. This will have a profound effect on you, maybe allowing you to move forward with your life for the first time since you were a child. It can be that liberating.

Hypnotic regression (going back in time) is an extremely powerful tool. Use it with caution. *Do not use it* if you are presently under the care of a mental health professional for a diagnosable mental illness. Check first with your therapist before you proceed and use it only with their permission. *Do not use it* if you have suffered severe trauma or if you are unable to control your emotions. The resulting emotional release may be more than you can handle without assistance from a properly trained therapist. You can find a credentialed psychologist well-trained in hypnosis by visiting the American Psychological Association's national referral network on the organization's website at www.apa.org.

WHY USE REGRESSION?

Ed came to me seeking help with uncontrollable diabetes. As I mentioned in an earlier chapter, diabetes often arises for people who have trouble digesting the sweetness of life. A quick conversation indicated this was very likely in Ed's case. He pushed himself hard, working nonstop and keeping his emotions at bay. He was cynical and didn't get much joy out of life. He had an especially tough case with his disease and had been unable to manage it with diet or medication.

Under hypnotic regression, Ed went to a time when he was a preschooler. Something had upset him, and he'd started crying. His father took him aside and very sternly upbraided him. "Be a man," his father said harshly. "Boys don't cry. Emotions are for women." Feeling intimidated by his father, Ed developed the attitude that it was whimsical and improper to *feel*. He needed to set his emotions aside and "be a man."

While still under hypnosis, Ed decided he didn't want to live like that any longer. He rejected the tough lesson his father taught him decades before and decided he could open himself to the sweetness of life. Sure enough, he started enjoying things—sunrises and sunsets, the taste of a meal, the pleasures of using his heart as well as his head. Not long after this session, his blood sugar levels fell into the normal range. He was able to quit his medication and keep diabetes at bay just by monitoring his diet.

For a number of good reasons, we aren't always able to make sense of a difficult experience when it happens. Children who encounter extreme difficulty simply aren't intellectually or emotionally mature enough to "sort things out." They need adult guidance and permission to work out their problems and don't always get it. Sometimes unaware, intolerant, or abusive family members, teachers, employers, or others prevent or prohibit us from working out our thoughts and feelings. Sometimes, trauma comes at us so fast and furiously that we only have time for crisis management. If a flood destroys your family home, all your effort would go toward survival with little or no time devoted to handling the traumatic stress. Or perhaps you've had the experience of setting aside your own emotional needs on the heels of tragedy in order to care for those you love, such as the teenager who quits school to go to work after his father dies so he can support the family.

For these and other valid reasons, we tend *not* to deal fully with the consequences of our difficult experiences. As a result, we push the distorted thoughts and feelings associated with painful or traumatic events down into the subconscious mind. Until we discover and release these distortions, they will sabotage our mental and physical health. Subconscious distortion will often set up a repetition compulsion—a repetitive pattern of flawed thought, feeling, and behavior that has dire consequences for health. In Ed's case, the distorted idea that "boys don't cry, emotions are for women" set up a lifelong revulsion for deep feeling of any kind. This distorted, repetitive compulsion created his diabetes and was making it worse.

Hypnotic regression will allow you to revisit your past to discover and release the subconscious distortion fueling your health problems. Like Ed, you will travel back in time, experience the source of old emotional pain and distorted thinking, and free yourself from it. Once liberated from the distortion, you will have the ability to reprogram the subconscious mind with distortion-free thinking and feeling consistent with your goals for a healthy, happy future.

WHAT TO EXPECT

Under hypnosis, I will invite you to go to a past time and place that will give you the insight and power you need for healing. Because the door to your subconscious mind is open and intuitive wisdom from the superconscious mind is available to you, your mind will naturally steer you to the right event(s). You won't have to think about it.

Remain passive and let your mind guide you. For example, you are probably aware of your difficult early life experiences and might naturally expect to go to one of these, but under hypnosis, your inner wisdom might take you to an event you previously considered trifling. Only when you experience this event under hypnosis do you see that it holds deep significance you overlooked at the time it happened.

Similarly, you might be hungry to revisit a trauma from childhood, one you've been trying to unravel for years, but your innate wisdom under hypnosis takes you instead to a time when life was very pleasant. I had a patient who had serious problems with anxiety and anger, and as a result, battled a formidable case of Irritable Bowel Syndrome (IBS). When she was regressed, she did not go back to the source of her anger. Instead, she went to a time when she had been extremely courageous, peaceful, and happy. This experience reminded her that she didn't need to be angry in the face of a threat. She embraced this feeling of courage and profound peace and was able to carry that feeling with her when she came out of hypnosis. Her IBS improved dramatically.

Under hypnosis, you may find yourself reliving a single event in unusual detail with uncanny accuracy, or you might take a whirlwind tour through a series of related events that have a shared theme. I remember one young man who went back to a difficult hospital stay when he was only two years old. During the regression, he saw a red-haired man standing nearby, talking with his father. After he left my office, he asked his parents about the man and they said, "Oh my goodness, we haven't seen that old friend in twenty years. How could you possibly remember him?" By contrast, I recall a beautiful, successful woman in her mid-thirties who came to me for help with painful uterine fibroid tumors. She had tried medication and had surgery twice to remove the tumors, but they kept coming back. In her first hypnotic regression, she surveyed her entire life: her father was overly critical, she learned to under-value herself as a child, and she preselected the men in her life to be just like her dad and underwent years of harsh treatment in important love relationships. Through these experiences, she became convinced she didn't measure up as a woman, a distortion that lodged symbolically in her reproductive organs. When she found this distortion, she released it. She went on to find the love she deserved with new optimism and her tumors shrank away.

History will present itself to you through a wide range of sensory and cognitive experiences. You may re-experience an event just as you lived it, seeing it through your eyes the way it happened at the time, accompanied by sensory awareness (sound, touch, smell, hearing, even taste). On the other hand, you may experience an event almost as though you were watching a movie, viewing it from outside yourself as a third-party observer. You could get extraordinary detail, or your experience might consist of somewhat indistinct images. Some people experience the past as thoughts about an event accompanied by mentally suggested imagery with no actual visual impressions. All of these types of experiences are valid, and all will deliver a powerful healing effect.

It is possible you'll see things with some level of distortion. You might experience a memory that you're certain isn't completely accurate. Such a distortion would occur if your father appears looking young and fit, sporting a head of thick black hair, when in real life your dad was much older, overweight, balding, and gray. A distortion of this type may be meaningless. On the other hand, sometimes the subconscious mind tries to make a point by changing history a little, adding features to the story, or inserting symbols into a memory sequence. For example, if you were born to your father late in his life and were ashamed of his advanced age and expanding waistline when you were a kid, the distortion above could have significance. Make note of these distortions when they arise. You can explore whether or not they have meaning both during and after the regression session.

Occasionally people experience an entire story that feels real but that you know never happened. Let's say there was a frozen pond near the house where you grew up, and under hypnosis you experience yourself falling through the thin ice on this pond—you might have drowned if your older brother hadn't jumped in to save you. You come out of hypnosis and think, "That didn't happen," but the experience seems so real. You decide to call your older brother and ask him about it. He says, "Are you on drugs? Of course it never happened." In this case, your subconscious mind made up the entire story to communicate something important to you. It therefore has metaphorical significance, and you should explore its meaning on this basis. A fantasy of this type might present itself if you felt as though you were always on "thin ice" with your parents when you were young and relied on your big brother for love and protection. Always remember that the subconscious mind loves to communicate through stories, symbols, and metaphors.

You may experience an obvious fantasy when you're regressed under hypnosis. A woman once came to me with bone spurs and severe pain in her feet and ankles. She was lesbian and had grown up with a lot of discrimination from her prominent Midwestern family. At college, she started to come out of the closet, pierced her body, and clothed herself in garb that said, "I don't belong here." She also discovered she was a luminous writer and a moderately good musician, but life after college involved working one mid-level clerical job after another. Under regression, this client experienced herself as a world famous rock and roll star. It was pure fantasy, but the effect of it was empowering. It encouraged her to come out publicly as a DJ at raves. She started to gain confidence. She went on to become a prominent, successful journalist, changed her wardrobe to something more traditional, and began to lead a comfortable upper middle-class life of the sort she would have had if she had never been persecuted for her sexual orientation. Meanwhile, the pain in her feet and ankles (which often occur when a person just doesn't want to be walking this earth) went away entirely.

On rare occasions, you might experience a fantastic, imaginative dream-like sequence under hypnosis. Let's say you find yourself flying on the back of a giant eagle. You're cruising at top speed through the Grand Canyon and you land on a mountain and see your dead grandfather standing there in the tasseled robes of a bishop with a serene smile on his face. This is an obvious fantasy, but you can bet it has strong metaphorical significance. Perhaps life was *really* tough when you were a kid and your grandfather was your only ally. He made you feel on top of the world, taught you about the meaning of life and to have faith in yourself and in God. The subconscious might offer you a fantasy of this type to remind you how powerful you are, how good life can be, and how much you loved your grandfather. You should anticipate profound levels of emotional release with this type of experience.

Regression is a thrilling and healing experience for most. Not always, though. The subconscious mind is capable of presenting a negative dream sequence. Frightening images could arise (running for your life through a haunted forest being chased by evil spirits, for example). These types of images might come if your subconscious is holding on to too much terror, which would be the case if you've been exposed to frightening events in real life and/or too many terrifying images (including too many horror movies). If this type of experience arises for you under hypnosis, just *shut it down.* You can stop any hypnotic experience just by saying to yourself, "No, I'm out of here." You can then choose to go on to another event or emerge yourself from the hypnotic session altogether by counting from one to five and opening your eyes. Working through negative subconscious imagery has the potential to provide deep levels of cathartic release from old fear, but you should *not* do it alone. To explore this type of experience under hypnosis, get help from a licensed therapist well-trained in hypnosis.

Maybe a quarter of the time, people will regress under hypnosis to a story that appears to be an alternative life script—a completely different life that seems to have occurred at some time in the distant past. This is the "past life" phenomenon, of which there has been a great deal written, beginning with Dr. Brian Weiss's groundbreaking book *Many Lives, Many Masters*. The idea of reincarnation is gaining acceptance in the West. According to a recent poll, about a third of all Americans believe in reincarnation, including more than 40 percent of people aged twenty-four to forty-five. In other parts of the world, reincarnation is already more fully accepted. There's no scientific proof for this. However, it is important for you to keep an open mind with regard to past life experience under hypnosis because of its potentially miraculous healing effect.

There is a scientific basis for past life phenomena that we touched on in chapter 3: the existence of subconscious archetypes, basic human personality patterns that we live out from deep inside the subconscious. These are personality roles like warrior, teacher, artist, caregiver, leader, seeker, and so on. A past life experience under hypnosis may indeed be a subconscious archetypal pattern expressing itself as an alternative life.

Let me share a true story that brings home just how powerful past life regression can be. Many years ago, a social worker named Mark came to see me. He was a born-again Christian diagnosed with Bell's palsy. Three years earlier, he'd been out on a lake in a boat. It got very cold, and as the winds whipped up, he became extremely chilled, particularly the left side of his face. While he was still out on the boat, he felt as though that part of his face was frozen. From that day on, he suffered partial paralysis and pain on that side of his face. It got progressively worse until the whole left side of his face and mouth drooped. His doctors tried a variety of medications and therapies, but nothing worked.

During hypnotic regression, Mark found himself in an unfamiliar place. At first, he thought he was in a subway tunnel but then realized he was on a concrete stairway in an underground military facility. He saw he was wearing a Nazi uniform and became aware that he was working as a guard (the warrior archetype) in a top-secret plant that was developing a nuclear bomb. He decided he couldn't be part of such a thing and made the decision to go AWOL. The facility was on an island in a cold northern sea. He caught a troop boat late at night and went back to the mainland, where he wandered, lost and weary, into the wilderness. He fell to the ground exhausted, went to sleep, and froze to death just before dawn—with the left side of his face frozen to the ice and snow.

When I brought Mark out of hypnosis, he touched his left cheek—and discovered he could feel the touch. He smiled broadly and the smile extended to both sides of his face. The left side of his face no longer sagged. In fact, his face had completely healed. He kept in touch with me for five years, letting me know that his face was still fine.

Remember, Mark was a born-again Christian. He didn't believe in the possibility of past lives. Was he really a German soldier in a previous life, or was he just experiencing an archetypal epic drama playing out in his subconscious mind? We cannot know. Research in this field has not evolved to the point of delivering an answer to that question. What we can know is that by accessing this "past life," my patient was immediately and permanently healed of his disorder. I see this in my work all the time. A majority of people who experience a "past life" under hypnosis will experience profound healing effects—psychological and/or physical. The healing occurs quite naturally once the metaphorical or archetypal "drama" is accessed and passed into consciousness from the subconscious mind. So never waste a good past life experience under hypnosis—it may have the potential to heal you dramatically.

There is one other type of experience you might have using hypnotic regression: a direct encounter with your super-conscious mind. Superconscious awareness is not fantasy. It is the actual experience of your own higher states of consciousness. It can vary strongly from person to person. Some common examples include the sense that you no longer have a physical body (but instead, a body of light or energy), super-human levels of peace, love and joy, a vastly expanded awareness (as if your mind has become large enough to embrace the earth and all that is in it), receiving personal insights (your purpose in life, why things have happened to you the way they have, which doctor to trust, and so on), or the ability to penetrate some of the mysteries of the universe. About 10 to 20 percent of people will have this type of experience early in their use of this method. You can expect the frequency of your super-conscious experience to grow, however, both in and out of hypnotic states, as you continue to use this method and the other methods in this book.

A Note of Caution

A small number of people who use hypnotic regression will experience a traumatic event that seems utterly real but that cannot be verified through their own conscious recollection, a witness, or any other objective source. There is such a thing as repressed memory that can be recovered under hypnosis. Memory obtained via hypnosis has figured prominently in some investigations and court cases, including cases of alleged sexual abuse.

Sometimes these memories are real and sometimes they are false. Except in cases where there is corroborating evidence that these events actually transpired, there is no scientific way to prove that these hypnotic recollections are accurate. However, real or not, they can be traumatic when they occur. If you use the hypnotic regression method in this chapter and experience what you believe to be a repressed memory of a traumatic event or events, you should work with a properly trained clinician. You need clinical expertise to sort out whether it is real or not and (in either case) deal with the consequences. If this happens to you, stop working with this method immediately and seek professional help.

The Method

Hypnotic regression is an extremely powerful tool that usually evokes strong emotional release, penetrating self-insight, and a sense of awe. You will want to give yourself some extra time with this method, including some time to decompress afterward. Including time for a little reflection, you'll need to set aside about ninety minutes to use the method.

Download Induction Gamma-V from www.miraculoushealthbook.com to begin. Burn this onto a CD and set up the room the way you have for the other hypnotic exercises. If you want to have a record of your experience, you may also want to set up a tape recorder nearby. This would allow you to describe your experiences aloud while under hypnosis and reflect on the contents of the tape later. Speaking aloud during this process will actually serve to deepen the experience for you.

Now play the download. In it, I will take you through five steps. The first step is an induction, with which you are now quite familiar.

The second step is called a *bridge*. It involves a series of suggestions and imagery designed to move your attention away from where you are right now and into a different time and place (a bridge across time or space). I might suggest, for example, that you imagine yourself floating up from where you are and then down into another time and place. Remember, to avoid steering yourself to anything in particular. Take a passive stance and let your mind lead you to your destination.

The third step is called *grounding*. You'll hear me ask you a series of questions that help "ground" you in the new place and time. These will be questions such as, "Is this place dark or light? Are you outside or inside? What are you wearing?" As you move through these grounding questions, more and more of your attention will focus on the time and place you are visiting, and it will become clearer to you. You will also remain aware of yourself in the present. I taught a luncheon seminar on hypnotic regression at a tony Washington, D.C., restaurant two years ago. At the end of the seminar, I took the owner of the restaurant into hypnotic regression. She went to the experience of dancing in a gold and silk gown at a palace ball in France in the 1700s. As she moved through the experience, she also deftly fielded questions from the patrons in the restaurant. As in her case, you'll go somewhere else but also stay home in the present.

Step number four is the *regression experience* itself. After I ground you in it, I will let you experience an event or series of events for a few minutes. During this time, if you've set up a tape recorder, you will want to share your experience aloud for future reference. Next, I will bridge you to a different event or series of events and then ground you in yet another experience from the past. After I let you spend several minutes experiencing whatever your mind presents to you, we will repeat the entire process one more time. In total, you will have three distinct excursions into a different time and place. Go wherever your thoughts take you on this guided tour. You will find important messages at every stop.

Once you've made these three journeys, I will ask you—while you're still in a deep hypnotic state—what these experiences were designed to teach you. In all likelihood, given what you know about the workings of the subconscious and super-conscious minds and about the symbolic presentation of disease, the answers will come quite easily. Finally, I will ask you how, based on what you now know, you plan to be different after this. How will you change your *story behind the story* based on what you've discovered? After this comes the fifth step where I help you *emerge* from the hypnotic state.

When you come out of hypnosis, spend some time writing about what you experienced and what you learned, even if you chose to tape record your observations during the session. You'll want to return to these notes from time to time and compare your experience from one regression session to another.

WHERE TO TAKE IT FROM HERE

Hypnotic regression work can generate unbelievably powerful healing. I estimate that two-thirds of the people who come to me with chronically debilitating problems or life-threatening illnesses get dramatically better from hypnotic regression work. It has the power to knock out bodily illness. Your experience may not be as dramatic as some of the experiences I've shared in this chapter (where one session resulted in complete recovery), but your experience will be nonetheless remarkable if you stay with the method. It will deliver results.

I suggest you try this method four times with one week between each session. The power of the method grows with each application, and most people need a series of four sessions to attain sufficient depth of exploration. Our emotions are many-layered, and one or two sessions will probably not allow you to penetrate deeply enough into your *story behind the story*. For example, let's say you have migraines and in an initial hypnotic session connect with old anger as the source of your headaches. In the next session, you probe deeper and discover there is great fear underneath your anger. In the session that follows, you uncover a well of sadness related to your fear, and so on. A series of four sessions should help you break sufficient mental ground to achieve measurable, meaningful changes in your mental and physical health—enough to get you jazzed about your future—and, in this example, enough to get rid of your migraines.

This technique is very, very powerful. It has the ability to provide you with wondrous levels of release from old pain or confusion and grant extraordinary insight into your nature and your own unique path in life. Owing to its power, it's best to wait a week between uses so you can effectively analyze and internalize the many revelations that are likely to come your way. More frequent use of the method could "swamp" you with new understanding and cause unnecessary confusion.

You'll always get a chance to go back to it, though. After your "introductory series," you will want to continue using hypnotic regression. I will help you decide how to build this method into your personal long-term plan for miraculous health in the final chapter of this book.

CHAPTER 11

ENERGY HEALING

When my children were growing up, we used to go to a family camp for a week at the end of the summer. Whole families (rather than just the kids) would stay in a bungalow and do all the camp activities. I quickly got the reputation of "camp healer." Every summer for five consecutive years, kids and adults alike would come to me with all kinds of minor ailments, everything from headaches to upset stomachs to sprained ankles. The camp nurse and the doctor on call really had very little to do because I could quickly heal problems without medication using energy healing—the ability to focus BioEM energy on a wound or illness to effect healing.

Most of the ailments I dealt with were simple things, but one evening I faced a truly serious situation. An eleven-year-old boy severed the tip of his finger while closing a Ping-Pong table. His family rushed him off to the hospital where doctors reattached it, but the prognosis was grim. The doctors could not be sure whether the reattachment would work, and they felt sure the finger would not function properly, even under a best-case scenario.

The boy returned to the camp heavily dosed with narcotics. Fingertips have a lot of nerve endings, so finger injuries are extremely painful. Despite the use of painkillers, this young boy was in agony—experiencing pain at a level of ten on a one-to-ten scale. He'd been like that for hours, and was trying to be tough, but his face and tears betrayed how excruciating this was for him. I went to work immediately, super-loading his finger and hand with BioEM energy. Within a matter of minutes, I dropped the pain from a ten to a two. Everyone was stunned how quickly we made progress, and the boy was utterly transformed—he finally felt human again.

I knew we'd only achieved the first step by getting the bulk of the pain out of the way. The critical next step was to make sure the finger would function fully once the tissues healed. I taught the boy how to focus his attention on his finger as a means to move energy into it. He was so encouraged by the instant progress we had just made on his extreme pain that he committed to getting the rest of the job done. He worked on his finger for a number of months and the finger ended up absolutely fine with full motion, strength, and sensation restored.

Energy healing has that kind of power. As you can see from this story, it's so simple even a child can do it.

THE MIRACULOUS POWER OF BIO-ENERGY

To understand how energy healing works, let's reflect on some of the wisdom in earlier chapters. As we discussed in chapter 2, your body possesses the inherent knowledge required to heal itself; every single cell of the body contains the intelligence required to recreate the entire body, let alone heal a particular problem. However, when you are stressed, exhausted, injured or ill, bodily energy stores become badly diminished. The body's innate intelligence cannot work because there is insufficient fuel to drive the process of healing. It's a bit like having a new Lexus in the driveway that's out of gas—all that intelligent engineering and design go to waste without fuel.

Recall also from chapter 2 that thought directs energy fields. Thought itself exists as subtle electromagnetic energy. You can use different ways of thinking to direct and focus BioEM energies to heal an illness or injury.

With these two concepts, you have two parts of a three-part healing strategy. The third part is that you need an energy source to draw on—and you have one. As I mentioned in chapter 6, energy flows into the body through the brainstem, the medulla oblongata located at the base of your head. You have the power, through directed thought, to draw in vast amounts of energy through this energy "portal" in the brain and send it into your body to effect healing.

The Method

I'm going to teach you a simple and highly effective method for energy healing that I use in my own work. It involves focusing your thought and attention to channel BioEM energy into your body or to a part of your body that is ill, injured, or in pain. We will also utilize the power of the breath to increase energy flow. In doing so, we'll be using a method that many athletes understand and employ. When Serena Williams takes a backhand whack at a tennis ball, she focuses all her concentration on the ball and blows out her breath in a burst to increase the amount of thrust (energy) behind the racket. If you work out at the gym under the guidance of a trainer, you already know the method. Let's say you're doing a bicep curl: you focus all your mental awareness on the bicep. You breathe in when you're relaxing the muscle and thrust the breath out when you contract the muscle to raise the dumbbell. Consequently, you super-charge that bicep with energy. Any weightlifter will tell you that doing bicep curls with this method is dramatically better than what you can achieve without it.

The method is easy. You can practice it now as you read these instructions. First, draw in a breath. As you do, put your awareness at the base of your head and imagine energy flowing inward. At the point where the indrawn breath pauses, focus your attention on the location of your physical problem (an organ, a joint, or even your entire body if that's the nature of your illness). Now push your breath out, and as you do, imagine the captured energy flowing into that part of your body. That's the method, start to finish.

You can tailor this method to suit your learning style and goals for healing. For example, feel free to imagine energy flowing into the body with the indrawn breath in any way that works for you. The indrawn breath creates a vacuum or "pull" inward. When you feel that pull, all you have to do is "think" energy is flowing into the back of your head, and it will. Visual, creative types might prefer to imagine a cloud of white light flowing into the base of the head as they draw in a breath. Any combination of these or similar techniques will allow you to take in huge amounts of energy for healing (more than you need actually).

The same holds true for the exhaled breath and how you focus it. You might need to focus energy on your heart, other internal organs, a bum knee, or if you have a system-wide problem (such as diabetes, Lyme disease, or metastasized cancer), the whole body. As you exhale, as long as you are concentrating your awareness on the location of your illness or injury, you will get the job done. As you push your breath out just "think" that energy is flowing into the body (or to specific body parts, as appropriate). Or, you can "imagine" energy flowing or washing into the area of the body in need of healing. Some people send the energy "through" the body, and others stream the energy "laser-like" from their head directly to afflicted areas. Still others "place" the energy in the body instantaneously (like the transporter on Star Trek—one moment the energy is in your head and the next moment it has arrived at its destination). Any one or a combination of these or similar techniques will work. As long as you are concentrating your attention on your illness or injury, the energy will flow to the appropriate location.

After practicing this method, you will be able to move extraordinary amounts of energy for healing. When I do energy-healing work on another person, I use this method to draw in energy and then pump it through my hands to focus it on that person's body, precisely as I described in exercise 2 of chapter 2.

The great thing about this method is that you can use it anytime, anywhere to great effect. A dose-response relationship applies to this method. This means that regular, small doses (such as those used by the boy at the beginning of this chapter) will deliver results, even if your problem is severe. So use it anytime, anywhere. Perhaps you have a few minutes while you're waiting for a meeting to start or standing in the checkout line at the grocery store. You can do this exercise with your eyes open without anyone else knowing what you're doing. With practice, you can use the method while you're moving about during the day with no loss of ability to keep pace with what's going on around you.

Because this method involves focusing your awareness, it is especially effective if you do it under hypnosis or during meditation. Under either of these two states, your focus is keen, your mind is calm, and there is nothing to distract your attention. I've provided a hypnotic process that guides you through this method at the end of this chapter.

WHAT TO EXPECT

By practicing this method, you will actually be able to perceive energy flowing into the back of your head and into your body. You might experience a slight sense of euphoria because of all the excess energy you're pumping through your mind. You will also experience noticeable improvements in your body right away. For example, your arthritic knee should feel noticeably less painful and have more mobility after five minutes of energy healing work.

How quickly you heal with this method will depend on two factors. The first is the severity of your affliction. You can relieve a headache in a few minutes, but it could take you three months of daily work to reverse a serious advanced orthopedic problem like osteoporosis. Even if your problem is serious, though, you will notice along the way that you're making progress. Embrace this progress and use it to keep going as long as necessary.

The other factor that will determine the speed of your recovery is the degree to which you are moving in tandem with your *story behind the story*. Energy healing provides significant results. However, the results are exponentially stronger—and lasting—if you do this work at the same time as you work with your *story*, making consistent gains in understanding yourself. The combination will make sustainable improvements to your health and wellbeing.

Under certain circumstances, energy-healing work can increase pain in the short run. A short-term increase in pain using this method is a sign of healing, not an indication that something is wrong. This happens because of something known as the "pain/healing paradox."

The basis for the pain/healing paradox is one we've mentioned before: insufficient energy in the nerves will dampen your ability to feel pain or even block out pain all together. If you get a gash on your arm, the doctor gives you a shot of local anesthetic to deaden the nerves in that area and it becomes numb. Then he stitches you up, and you don't feel a thing until the anesthetic wears off—then it hurts. When energy flow stops, the pain stops. When energy flow is restored, pain returns. You see this paradox at work with spinal cord injuries or other cases where the nervous system is seriously compromised: in the immediate term paralysis or severe numbness results and the sensation of pain is dampened or absent altogether. When surgery or therapy restores the flow of energy to the nervous system, the sensation of pain returns. This type of pain is a sign of progress; it's a sign that energy flow has been restored to deadened tissues.

The mind is capable of performing a function similar to chemical painkillers and anesthetics. In cases of chronic acute pain, the mind will act to withdraw energy from the nerves in the afflicted area so the pain will go down. This reaction of the mind is helpful in the short term. Acute pain makes it difficult to function and can create problems in other parts of your body. For example, a person who has severe arthritic pain in her hips might naturally accommodate her pain by leaning forward, keeping her lumbar spine too rigid and putting too much stress on her knees. Over time, she's likely to end up not only with bad hips but also a bad back and knees. Therefore, the tendency of the mind to withdraw energy from the nerves is good because it helps avoid these additional complications. The problem is that when energy flow is reduced over a long period, bodily tissues become deadened and healing potential is reduced.

Energy-healing work increases energy flow. It has the effect of decreasing pain 90 percent of the time. In cases where the flow of energy in the body has been strongly dampened over a long period, however, use of this method may cause an increase in pain as energy begins to "enliven" deadened tissues. If this happens to you, know that the pain is temporary and will go away with continued energy healing work. Typically, this will even happen over the course of one treatment session where the pain rises at the start and then lessens by the end, though it sometimes lasts over several sessions.

Energy-healing work *cannot* be harmful. Regardless of the level of early-stage discomfort you feel, your healing will be considerably faster with energy work than it would be with traditional medicine alone. In fact, as with the boy with the severed finger, healing can come with energy work in cases where *no* healing is possible through traditional means like chemical painkillers.

Energy-healing work can bring you comfort quickly and has a tremendous impact on healing over time. It can even help you keep your dreams alive. I had a patient who was a teacher throughout her career, but her real love was volleyball. She played in a competitive league that culminated in a national championship every year. Her ultimate goal was to win a championship game.

She reached a point where she retired from teaching, but she was still a competitive volleyball player, and the game acquired an even more significant place in her life as a result. By this time, she was nearing sixty and most of the people in her league were half her age. She started getting injured regularly. After every game, she'd be nursing a twisted knee, a bruised elbow, or strained neck with too little time to recover before the next match. Her ailing body was forcing her to retire from the game, and this caused her great despair.

I did energy-healing work on her regularly and taught her how to work on herself. She employed the methods religiously. After a match, she'd limp off the court and start healing her injury of the week. By the end of the season, her team had made it to the championships and she was in better shape than she'd been in years. Just prior to the championship game, she redoubled her use of the method. The next week, she came in to see me, proudly sporting her gold medal. She was as integral to the victory as the "youngsters" on her team.

ENERGY HEALING UNDER HYPNOSIS

You can get dramatic results using this method under hypnosis, when your mental clarity and focus are many times greater than in a normal waking state.

To use the method under hypnosis, download Induction Gamma VI from www.miraculoushealthbook.com, burn it onto a CD, and set up the room in the same way you have for previous hypnotic exercises. Now start the download. I'll move you through a hypnotic induction and then guide you through the method (drawing energy in through the medulla oblongata during the in-breath and directing the energy into the body with the out-breath).

First, we'll use the method to cleanse and strengthen every energy center in your body. This is the equivalent of giving your body a tune-up—I'll help you make sure your energy centers are working as optimally as possible.

Next, I'll guide you through use of the method to target the illness in your body. If your physical problems manifest throughout your body (certain blood disorders, systemic infections, diabetes, leukemia, metastasized cancer, and so on), take this time to radiate every cell in your body with energy. If you need to focus on a particular part or parts of the body (heart, stomach, an injured hip, for example) center your attention there.

Concentrate on one area per session. This can be a combination of body parts if they are in the same location—say your left shoulder and left arm. However, if you have pain in distinct areas—say your left shoulder and right knee—it's best to run the download twice, concentrating on a different area each time.

After you've spent several minutes targeting specific illness or injury in your body, I will guide you through a process for saturating the entire body with energy. Then I will emerge you from hypnosis.

FREQUENCY OF USE

Energy healing work should be a daily part of your personal healing regimen. Use it as often as you can. Do it for a few minutes before you end each meditation and in mini-healing doses throughout the day. Set aside the time to do it twice a week under hypnosis using the method I've provided here. You'll love the impact this has on your body and—since you'll be tuning up your energy centers at the same time—your overall wellbeing.

CHAPTER 12

THE GEARSHIFT EXERCISE

Over the course of this book, we have discussed the four levels of mind—the conscious, subconscious, individual super-conscious, and universal super-conscious. Various exercises you've worked with so far have allowed you to touch on one or several of these. Now, I'm going to introduce you to an exercise that will allow you to experience *all* of them. I hope you're ready for one of the biggest adventures of your life.

The method in this chapter allows you to "cruise up" through the four levels, harnessing ever-greater degrees of mental power as you go. I call it the Gearshift Exercise because it's like driving a Ferrari, going from zero to sixty in less than five seconds and then accelerating even faster (fortunately, there are no speed limits on this highway).

The Gearshift Exercise is the most powerful of the methods provided in this book. While you shouldn't use it alone (it's critical that you use all the tools that help you explore your *story behind the story*), it can make a dramatic difference—maybe the essential difference—in your ability to achieve miraculous health. Two years ago, a middle-aged woman with multiple sclerosis (MS) came to see me for help with depression. She had recently left a marriage of twenty-five years to a man who'd abused her emotionally, though in public he was an icon of service to her community and her church. This woman had no remarkable problems early in life. She'd grown up in a loving, stable family in northern

California. She stayed in her abusive marriage for so long because her family and religious values would not let her walk away. However, two and a half decades of "closet" abuse had left her emotionally and spiritually scarred. Her MS worsened considerably, to the point that she was having trouble walking and concentrating and was in danger of losing her job as a teacher.

Over a few months, we used hypnotic regression work, energy healing, meditation, and talk-therapy to restore her self-esteem and optimism. Through this, she realized her *story behind the story* was to discover and live out her dreams, rather than fulfill the expectations of her parents, church, and community. She came into a deeper, more authentic contact with God that renewed her faith. Her depression lifted entirely and her concentration improved somewhat. She didn't make significant progress with the MS, though, until I taught her the Gearshift Exercise.

Once she started doing the Gearshift, she noticed an improvement in her walking. Soon, she actually started to do a little ballroom dancing, something she had enjoyed in her youth. Three months into this, she came to my office, smiling ear to ear. She'd just been to her doctor, who told her—astonished—that the scar tissue near her brainstem (an indicator of MS) was now gone. It was no longer "observable."

Clearly, all the methods we used helped in this woman's recovery—even the ballroom dancing. However, the Gearshift Exercise made the crucial difference. It was able to effect physiological change when the other methods could not.

WHAT YOU CAN USE IT FOR

The Gearshift Exercise is designed to activate all four levels of mind to work together to accomplish any noble goal in life; it increases the "power of positive thinking" more than a hundredfold because with it you have the ability to call the Universe into action on your behalf.

If you suffer from physical injury or illness, you can use the Gearshift Exercise to heal yourself. You can also use it to change events in the world around you to achieve any goal related to your *story behind the story* or any personal aspiration, to heal others, or contribute to the social good. For example, let's say you have a string of unhappy relationships behind you, and you discover that your *story behind the story* is compelling you to learn how to love and be loved unconditionally. You could use the Gearshift Exercise to attract a great love in your life.

There are some important limitations on the use of this method however. You can't use it to skirt your lessons, override the free will of another person, or cause harm. These agendas run counter to the innate virtue of super-conscious mind; it will always act to heal and liberate, to bring you into honest authentic relationship with your *story behind the story*, and will *never* abrogate another's free will.

What does this mean in practical terms? Let's say you want to attract greater love in your life but are now involved in an unhappy marriage. You could use the Gearshift Exercise to focus on improving your marriage—that would be noble. In this case, you could expect to see *a lot* of change in *your* ability to love and be loved. However, if your spouse decides *not* to change, the Gearshift Exercise will not override his or her free will.

The super-conscious mind operates on the principle of unlimited abundance. The Gearshift Exercise gives you a means to tap into this abundance and get it working for you. In the Psalms, it is written, "Delight in the Lord and He'll grant you the desires of your heart." Though the terminology here is exclusively religious, the principle is accurate and universal: the super-conscious mind is extravagantly generous. You simply have to know how to "think" or commune with it on its own terms. The Gearshift Exercise will let you do that. My clients, who represent all walks of life and all cultural, philosophical, and religious perspectives, have used it to gain everything from physical health to an increase in income so they can afford to pay their medical bills, and a whole lot more.

BE CAREFUL WHAT YOU ASK FOR

The Gearshift Exercise is so effective you'll want to think carefully about what you desire before you employ it. For example, take a man I've been working with over the last four years. He came up hard in New York. He could never win his father's love and never felt like he amounted to anything. He didn't have much culture, income, or education. Then he married a woman who belittled him. His children didn't understand him either, though he loved his family very much. All this lost love and lack of self-esteem caused significant depression, along with excessive weight gain and circulatory problems that threatened his life.

As we worked with the methods in this book, he came to understand that his *story behind the story* was compelling him to love and respect himself. His depression cleared. His health improved, but as part of his quest to make justice for himself, he decided that he really wanted to have a nice, big house to enjoy with his family. His desire was not entirely superficial. After having too little in life, he wanted the American Dream, and his desire was not selfish.

When he started working with me, he was making about $50,000 a year doing work that he despised. I taught him how to do the Gearshift Exercise, and now he's clearing more than a million annually, doing work that he loves. He achieved his dream through the power of this method, and he's using his newfound wealth to help others. Recently, he met a poor family, found employment for the father, and bought the father a car because he knew that transportation would make the difference in the family's survival. After Hurricane Katrina, he bankrolled emergency response missions to New Orleans and went along to help distribute supplies to the flood victims. He's a good man. He's a hero in his own way.

However, his financial success has come at a cost. He's always on the go. He has the beautiful house, but he is seldom home to enjoy it with his family.

This method can bring you what you want—just be sure that you really want it.

THE SCIENCE BEHIND THE METHOD

Before I explain the method, let's review our model of "mind" as a means to reconsider all that you are and what you are capable of being. The wisdom from previous chapters is summarized in the following list and table:

- Your body and everything else in existence is made of energy, and energy is governed by thought.
- You are "thinking" at four distinct levels of mind—you are simply unaware of it.
- You have to become *aware* of your thought at any one level of mind in order to harness the ability to move energy at that level.

	LEVEL 1	LEVEL 2	LEVEL 3	LEVEL 4
SCIENTIFIC TERM	Conscious mind	Subconscious mind	Individual super-conscious mind	Universal super-conscious mind, also the unified field
COMMON TERM	Ordinary self	Deep, also hidden self	The soul	God
TYPE OF THOUGHT	Analysis, also logic	Symbolic, also metaphoric	Intuitive	Meditative
GEAR	First	Second	Third	Fourth

The vast majority of people are only aware of their conscious mind—the smallest, weakest part of the mind. This is the first gear in the Gearshift Exercise.

If you've been practicing the methods in this book, you have most certainly experienced the second gear, the subconscious mind. This is a realm of metaphorical and symbolic thinking—the deepest sense of self, life purpose, and meaning. It is two to three times the size and power of your conscious mind and is exerting a substantial influence on your health.

Consistent work with the methods may also have allowed you to glimpse the third gear, individual super-consciousness, or soul awareness. This level of mind relies on intuitive thought to understand and influence the electromagnetic energy fields associated with your mind and body, as well as with other people, places, and events.

If you have encountered fourth gear, universal super-consciousness, you would certainly be aware of it. It has one very specific attribute: a profound peace that deepens into "bliss"—an expansive, ever-new joy that keeps growing without end. We access universal super-consciousness (God) via meditative thought, which allows us to experience ourselves as part of the infinite intelligence in the quantum (subatomic) energy field that creates and sustains the entire universe.

Your ability to "think" at all four levels will determine the character and power of your BioEM field, which is radiating energy through your body and out into the world. Your BioEM field is interacting with the energy fields associated with your body's internal organs and processes, where it fosters either wellness or illness. Your field is also interacting with the energy fields associated with other people, places, and things. It has the ability to determine your moment-to-moment experience, shape your destiny, and have an impact on other people and events. At this level, your field can effect changes in the world around you that will determine how you are living out your *story behind the story*. Your BioEM field also interacts with the universal quantum field, which has the ability to bring you into extravagant levels of enlightened wisdom, peace, and joy. Even the briefest encounter with the quantum field (God) will result in an instantaneous benefit to your physical, mental, and spiritual health.

Imagine what you could accomplish if you could harness all this mental power. The Gearshift Exercise helps you do just that.

THE METHOD

During the Gearshift Exercise, we will be combining hypnosis with meditative techniques, so if you don't know how to meditate or haven't been meditating, go back to chapter 4 and familiarize yourself with the basic meditation technique described there before you proceed.

To experience the Gearshift Exercise, download induction Gamma-VII from www.miraculoushealthbook.com and burn it onto a CD. Set aside time, ensure your privacy, and prepare your room as you have for the other hypnotic exercises.

Before you start the download, consider what it is you want to accomplish with the method. It can be any noble desire: perfect health, better medical care, a nice home, a great love relationship, a fantastic job, freedom from debt, a strong family, coming into peace and joy—whatever fits your goals based on your needs and your *story behind the story*. Just be sure to have a clear, focused idea of what you want to achieve before you use the method. If you come into the method with multiple or ill-defined objectives you will not be able to gain the benefit. You can have multiple goals but you'll want to focus on one goal every time you use the method.

Recall the universal principle of abundance and don't think "small" with regard to your goals. Don't think for a moment that you'll have to settle for anything less than what you desire. Think big.

Now you're ready to start. Turn on the CD. In it, you will hear me guide you through an induction. Then I will have you meditate for a few minutes until you are very calm. Next, I'll invite you to think about your goal from the perspective of ordinary logic and reason (first gear) for three to five minutes. I'll invite you to think about all the good reasons why you should get to your goal. During this time, any number of things might occur to you about your goal that hadn't occurred to you before. If you are in need of surgery, for example, it might occur to you to call an old friend from college who's on the surgical staff at a major hospital for a trustworthy reference. At this stage, be aware that your thoughts are radiating into the world like a radio broadcasting tower, affecting the subatomic structure of matter around you, to draw one preferred outcome out of the quantum (subatomic) energy fields related to your issue.

After you've done this for a few minutes, I will ask you to return to meditation as a means to restore your mental peace and focus. Then we'll move on to second gear. I will guide you, via direct suggestion, into the use of imagery to help you create a mental movie of how you can go from where you are to where you want to be. I will leave you at this level of exploration for three to five minutes. During this time, the power of your subconscious mind will work on helping you achieve your goal. At the end of this gear, I will have you ask your subconscious mind to present to you a symbol of what you are seeking. Be open to whatever you receive.

You might or might not receive a definite visual symbol. Last year, I was guiding an elderly woman through the Gearshift. She was using it to heal her husband. They were on the brink of retirement, and he was suffering from pulmonary hypertension, which had slowed him down a good bit. His illness had made him hidebound, rigid, and unhappy and threatened their dream of an easy retirement. As she worked this stage of the Gearshift, she saw a lock springing open, symbolizing to her that he was being freed from his resentment. You may not get a visual symbol like this; you may get color, sound, even smell, or just a strong feeling. If you get nothing, do not be alarmed. It means that your subconscious already delivered its message during the first three to five minutes of second gear and has nothing more to say right now.

I will next direct you to meditate for a few minutes to acquire a deeper and more expanded state of awareness. After that, I'll guide you into third gear—individual super-consciousness—using imagery. Once you're there, I'll invite you to affirm the rightness and goodness of your goal, with statements like, "This is mine for the asking. I deserve it. The universe wants this for me. I have it *now*." This type of thought equates with intuitive, direct, immediate "knowing" that your goal is as good as achieved. As you do this, be aware that your mental energies are radiating out into the world to cause the energy fields related to your issue to conform to your will.

I will let you remain in individual super-consciousness for about ten minutes. Sometimes, while people are doing their affirmations in third gear, they slip back into second or first gear and start doubting themselves with thoughts like, "Can I really do this? Could this really be working? I'll never get better." If this happens to you, just realize that you've slipped out of third gear. Shift away from negative thinking immediately. Just kick it out and go back to that imagined deep immediate feeling of knowing, "I have this; it is mine."

I will then direct you to meditate for a few minutes in order to prepare for entry into fourth gear—universal super-consciousness. Here, you will not focus on your goal anymore. You will focus on merging into the totality of the universal quantum field, or Spirit. Universal mind already knows what you need and desire. Merging into union with this level of mind will naturally "lock it in." I will leave you in this state of vastly expanded awareness for several minutes, and then I'll emerge you from hypnosis.

That's the Gearshift Exercise. I promise it will blow your mind.

How Often to Use It

I urge you to practice this exercise over an extended period. Start by using it every three days for a couple of weeks to focus on your most critical needs (like bodily health). Observe the amount of power and change it delivers. As your health improves, you can begin to pursue important goals related to your *story behind the story*—the things you need to live out your *story* more authentically (more courage and less fear or anger, or a better love in your life, and so on). After that, you can use it to pursue any noble desire whatsoever.

When used in concert with the other methods in this book, the Gearshift Exercise can literally change your life. Set your sights high here. Dream bigger than you thought it possible to dream. Imagine your highest, noblest goals and make it your intention to achieve those goals. You have the right to make your dreams come true—now you have the tool you need to make it happen.

PART FOUR

SUPPLEMENTAL METHODS

CHAPTER 13

COGNITIVE REPROGRAMMING

A s we've discussed, unresolved emotion creates dis-ease in the mind that transfers to the body in predictable ways to create and sustain physical illness. Negative emotions not only rob us of joy in life but also play a significant role in our health problems. That means negative emotions have to go.

In this section of the book, I will describe several psychotherapeutic tools that you can use to release negative emotions and speed your healing process. You will want to rely on one or several of these tools as part of your own customized treatment plan, which I will help you to develop soon.

AS YOU THINK, SO SHALL YOU FEEL

If you're a hands-on kind of person, you are going to love the cognitive reprogramming method described in this chapter. It is brief, and after you learn how to do it, you won't need my help to apply it. You can use it anytime, anywhere, and if used consistently, you will feel dramatically better in just three to four weeks.

The method I am going to teach you comes from cognitive therapy, a branch of traditional psychotherapy that is responsible for most of the advances in the field of psychology over the last thirty years. Aaron T. Beck, MD, first introduced cognitive therapy to the field of psychology in the 1960s. Beck believed that understanding the way people perceive and interpret experiences (known as cognition) was the key to freeing them from unhealthy emotional patterns.

Beck focused initially on depressed clients, ultimately expanding his research to cover other forms of mental disharmony. He discovered that "errors" in people's thinking caused and perpetuated their emotional disease. Errors in thought arise from numerous sources: experiences you had in your family of origin, social milieu, school, personal relationships, and other influences that introduce some level of distortion in your thinking. Beck developed cognitive therapy as a means to discover the "distorted" or "unrealistic" thinking that drives a person's negative feelings and behaviors.

Cognitive therapy has evolved a lot over the four decades since Beck's groundbreaking research. The core notion behind it remains the same, however: feeling follows thought. People who suffer chronically from negative emotions (anger, fear, resentment, powerlessness, poor self-esteem) suffer from a distorted thought process. If you can discover and correct the distortion in thought, the negative emotions disappear. What you think defines how you feel. How you were thinking last year affects how you feel today. What you think today will determine how you feel tomorrow. Your thoughts are not just a reaction to your immediate experience. They have a historical genesis (what you were taught to think years ago) and program how you are going to feel and react to your experience in the future.

This concept is liberating and should inspire a great deal of optimism about yourself and the human species. If you think accurately in any situation you find yourself, even if it's a difficult situation, strong emotions will not overwhelm you. Moreover, you won't find a disparity between your expectations and your experience, and therefore, you will not feel badly stressed.

When I introduce my clients to this concept, many agree with it. However, some will say "No way, Doc. When I'm swamped by bad feelings, I'm not thinking at all—the feelings just rise up out of nowhere. I'm not thinking; I'm just feeling." Certainly, that's how it seems when powerful emotion emerges, but the research is abundantly clear: thought is the governor of your emotions. Remember that you are always "thinking" at multiple levels: conscious thought is only the tip of the iceberg and most of what you're "thinking" is hidden from your awareness. When you feel smothered by powerful emotion, it's usually because distorted thinking in the subconscious mind has been churning away in secret. You are only aware of the negative emotion that follows and the negative effects it has on your mental and physical health.

There are many cognitive therapy methods, several of which are quite helpful. The method I teach here differs from the majority of approaches in one important way: it allows you to drill down into the subconscious mind to reprogram the distorted thought process there. The healing effects of this approach are rapid and extraordinary.

Many years ago, a successful middle-aged businessman came to see me for help. This man constantly suffered from colds, the flu, and viral infections of every sort. No sooner would he recover from one when another would assail him. His doctor could find no physical cause for it and referred him to me on the hunch that a psychological problem was fueling his repeated illness. When I met with the man, I found him to be extremely anxious and driven. For his entire adult life, he had worked a seventy-hour workweek. When most people would be on the brink of exhaustion, my client would find a burst of energy and stay at a task until completed, no matter what it took out of him. He didn't realize it, but he was literally working himself to death.

This man's father, a colonel in the army, had raised him under the strictest military expectations for performance in the face of adversity. His history made it clear that the focus of our work was to find and dismantle the distortions in his thought that compelled him to sacrifice his own essential need for rest.

For three sessions, we used hypnosis to uncover and release some of the difficult early life experiences that fueled this man's anxiety. I also taught him the cognitive reprogramming approach I describe in this chapter, which he used (not surprisingly) with military consistency. Shortly after we began our work together, he arrived one day in my office to say, "I've found the distortion in my thinking. The last time we were together, I told you I thought the cause for my anxiety was my work ethic and too much responsibility. You said 'those thoughts are accurate' and told me to look a little deeper. So I applied the cognitive reprogramming method again and found the distortion in my thinking that makes me feel like I'm going to explode if I don't keep working: I thought that I would be punished if I didn't make the grade."

It turned out that when my client was a boy, his father placed high demands on him and punished him severely if he failed to perform at that level. The boy's experience created a distortion in his thinking: "If I don't perform at the A-plus level *all* the time, there'll be hell to pay." So, he drove himself to be a superman, and this drive compromised his health. After he found this distortion and reprogrammed it, he eased back and moved into a phase of life that was self-loving, self-compassionate, and a whole lot healthier and happier—interestingly, with no loss in performance.

THE METHOD

The following simple cognitive reprogramming method can change the way you think at both the conscious and subconscious levels. It'll shift your feeling into peace, happiness, and a sense of personal potency. This, in turn, will improve your mental and physical health in dramatic ways.

The focus of this process is to target distortion in your thought process as it arises in response to specific events and challenges. You can use it any time you feel extreme emotional dis-ease.

The process has seven simple steps. As you gain familiarity with its use, you will be able to complete it in a couple of minutes. Near the end of this chapter, I summarize the steps in a seven-bullet "cheat sheet" you should carry in your pocket or purse for future reference.

STEP 1: BE AWARE OF WHAT YOU'RE FEELING IN THE MOMENT.

This method works best if you use it at the very point when you're feeling bad. If you have your antenna up, you'll catch negative emotion as it actually happens, but a lot of us move through the day without realizing how we actually feel until someone or something draws our attention to it. The first crucial step in this process is to stay aware and notice when you are starting to feel bad emotionally. If you aren't aware of it, you'll miss the opportunity to reprogram it altogether.

STEP 2: LABEL THE EMOTION(S) YOU'RE FEELING.

At the point when you realize you're feeling bad, take a few seconds to label your emotions. Is it anger, fear, sadness, frustration, shame, guilt, or some other emotion? You are now trying to understand what you're feeling, not what you're thinking. Some people have trouble distinguishing between the two, so it is important to your success that you can discern the difference. If your boss takes you down a peg in a meeting with your colleagues because you failed to get a job done, you might feel anxious, fearful, shamed, guilty, or angry. You might *think*, "I don't deserve this," or "He's being an ass," but that's not how you feel. As best you can, take note of how you're feeling. Early on, you might even want to write this down. As you keep using this method, you will be able to see patterns of emotional response to situations; this will deepen your self-awareness and your success with the method.

STEP 3: LOOK AT THE THOUGHTS BEHIND THE FEELING.

Now ask yourself, "What are my thoughts related to this feeling?" This step is usually as simple as looking at the thoughts moving in the back of your mind at that moment. Let's say the boss *has* embarrassed you publicly, and you're feeling very anxious. You start looking at the "thoughts" related to this feeling, and you find several. In addition to, "I don't deserve this," or "He's being an ass," you also may think, "My boss doesn't like me and has it in for me." Whatever you think, make a mental note of it, or if circumstances allow, write it down.

STEP 4: ASK YOURSELF "WHERE'S THE DISTORTION?"

At this stage, you're concerned with finding the distortion in your thinking. If you're feeling strong negative emotion moving through you, *assume* your thinking is distorted. Sometimes, you have to look hard for it. Consider our example: your boss has publicly embarrassed you, and you become very anxious and aware of three thoughts related to your anxiety ("I don't deserve this," "My boss is an ass," and "My boss doesn't like me and has it in for me"). Now you have to ask yourself, "Where is the distortion?" You may review your thoughts and conclude they are entirely accurate: you didn't deserve the harsh treatment (you are dedicated to your work and a productive employee overall), your boss is being an ass (only an angry selfish boss takes down a subordinate in front of his or her colleagues), and based on your boss's historical pattern of antagonism toward you, you conclude your boss really *does* have it in for you. All three of your initial thoughts on the matter appear to be accurate and free of distortion. In this case, you have to look deeper. Only a distorted thought will drive chronic emotional pain. Accurate thoughts, even if they point to a significant challenge on your horizon ("My boss has it in for me"), will not create chronic ill feeling.

Sometimes finding the thought distortion can be a little tricky. I remember a man who came to me a number of years ago, a brilliant young MD research scientist who was suffering from depression. He'd gotten into trouble by standing up to a very powerful superior who'd unfairly criticized him. After that, he experienced continuous difficulty at work. When I asked him to identify the thought behind his depression, he exclaimed, "I'm depressed because this powerful man is ruining my career!" I pushed him, saying, "Well, that thought is accurate. To find the source of your depression you have to go deeper." He pushed and pushed for two sessions and finally found it. Dropping his head into his hands, he said, "I've ruined my career just like my father ruined his." It ended up that at a similar age, his father had crossed his boss, and the boss went on a crusade to damage his father's reputation. The father's career eventually plummeted, leaving the family destitute. In the back of my client's mind was the distorted thought that his problems with his boss were going to ruin his future in the same way. When he realized the distortion, he let it go. He came to understand that he was a different person from his father; there was no basis in fact to assume his career was going to be ruined. The corrected distortion in his thinking freed him of his depression. He went on to make amends with his boss and subsequently achieved extraordinary levels of success in his field. Like my client, you may have to dig a little to discover the source of the distortion in your thinking.

STEP 5: CORRECT THE DISTORTION.
Once you've found the distortion, correct it with a simple "counter-claim" of undistorted truth. In the example I gave, my client corrected his distortion by thinking, "I am not my father. I can make things right with my boss. My career is not ruined." That correction freed my client from depression and unleashed the mental power he needed to remake his destiny. As you get good with this process, you will discover related patterns of distortion in your thinking and develop a series of "counter-claims," affirmations of truth that directly reverse these patterns. You might want to write out

these affirmations and use them whenever you discover a familiar distortion at work in your thinking.

STEP 6: HOW WOULD YOU FEEL IF YOU BELIEVED THE CORRECTION?

Now, begin to imagine how you'd feel if you believed the correction in your distorted thinking. This step will facilitate a shift in your feelings. You may still feel challenged but now hopeful, optimistic, confidant, and open to myriad possibilities for your future. You might even be happy and become aware of precisely what you should do to move forward to achieve your goals. Write down or make a mental note of these feelings and any details that arise in relation to them.

Some people have trouble with this step because they don't actually "believe" the corrected thought. The old distorted thought might tug at you, and you may want to cling to it out of habit. You are at a crossroads at this point. If you find yourself in a tug-of-war between an old distortion in your thinking and a new distortion-free idea, throw some good old-fashioned willpower into adopting the change. Realize you are attached to the old thought pattern because you've been brainwashed by the effects of memory and conditioning. Do you really want to remain attached to your conditioned distorted thoughts or would you rather adopt the new way of thinking and take control of your life? The old thought pattern needs to go if you are going to restore your freedom, dignity, and self-efficacy. Remind yourself you deserve this newfound freedom and power and stick with the process. The benefits will far outweigh the effort required to jettison the old way of thinking.

STEP 7: IMAGINE THE NEW FEELINGS FOR SIXTY SECONDS.

Whatever these new more positive feelings might be (optimism, confidence, happiness, and so on), repeat them to yourself with a strong sense of conviction for sixty seconds. Revel in the release of the old emotions and the delight and freedom associated with the new feelings and distortion-free thinking. Give it a full sixty seconds. You do not want to cut this step short. Remember that the "language" of the subconscious mind is imagery, metaphor, and deep feeling, so imagine yourself liberated by this new sense of who you are. During this step, you are broadcasting an advertisement to your subconscious mind—a new way of thinking and feeling that penetrates into the subconscious mind and reprograms the distortion that is lurking there.

YOUR PLAN FOR DEVELOPING SKILL WITH COGNITIVE REPROGRAMMING

Here is a brief summary of the cognitive reprogramming method:

- Be aware of what you're feeling.
- Label your feelings.
- Look at the thoughts behind your feelings.
- Ask yourself, "Where's the distortion?"
- Correct the distortion.
- Ask yourself how you'd feel if you believed the correction.
- Run the new feeling in your imagination for sixty seconds.

This seven-step summary is your cheat-sheet for the cognitive reprogramming process. Copy it down and put it in your pocket or purse for future reference. If you follow this method, you'll get amazing results.

If you implement this method a third of the time you find yourself gripped by a negative emotion and follow the method closely (no missed steps), you will find that negative emotions and the physical problems associated with them are noticeably better in just three to four weeks. Stay aware of your negative emotional states and you'll get the results you're looking for.

When you're first starting to use the method, until you get good at it, you'll want to dwell on the steps in depth and write down your observations. Life doesn't always allow for an intermission of this sort, but do what you can. If you're the maid of honor at your sister's wedding and feel intensely negative emotion in the middle of her vows, you aren't going to interrupt the service by whipping out a pad of paper and a pen. However, you might choose to stay in the parking lot for three minutes and jot a few things down before you drive on to the reception. Interestingly, many people are hit by powerful feelings while they're driving. It seems to be a natural time for reflection for many of us. My clients who use the cognitive reprogramming method to good effect sometimes pull off the road into a parking lot to work the process rather than miss a good opportunity to find the freedom that comes with this method.

Working this process may be a little challenging at first, but if you stay with it, it will become second nature and fall into place for you rapidly and powerfully. You will quickly be able to identify patterns of distortion in your thinking and quickly evolve a set of counter-claims (undistorted thoughts or affirmations) designed to reprogram them. In a matter of moments, you will be able to identify how you feel, know what you're thinking, find the distortion, counteract it with an affirmation of truth, understand how the new idea should make you feel, and imaginatively revel in the new feelings for sixty seconds. People who get good at this method can work it in two minutes without taking notes or creating a disruption in the flow of circumstances around them.

This hands-on method will deliver dramatic results that build your self-confidence. You'll be able to experience newfound health quickly and know that you achieved it through your own will and effort.

CHAPTER 14

CATHARTIC AND
EXPRESSIVE TECHNIQUES

S ome years ago, a man in his early fifties came to see me for anger management. In addition to his emotional issues, he suffered from degenerative disc disease that had created severe problems in his neck and
shoulders. He was hunched over and in a lot of pain, which made him
extremely irritable. His job was on the line because of his anger, and his
firm's human resource specialist had directed him to me for therapy.

This person was not so unlike many people who have legitimate gripes
in life. His father drank excessively when he was growing up. His mother
put a lot of pressure on him to be the man of the household and be a dad to
his little brother. He was never allowed to be a kid. As a young adult, he'd
married a woman who was a good bit like his mother and who put even
more pressure on him to perform. Life had abused this man, and he chose
to get angry in response to it. In fact he'd become so obnoxious and offen-
sive that no one wanted to listen to him. He had no one to talk to and had
repressed his feelings for more than three decades. By the time he walked
into my office, he was like a dormant volcano on the verge of exploding, to
the point that he was a danger to himself and others.

Over two months of weekly therapy with me, this man poured out his
life story. By the end of the two months, he was no longer angry. He'd just

really needed to vent his feelings. In the few sessions that followed, I used hypnosis and talk-therapy to help him come fully to grips with his *story behind the story* and move into peace. As he did this, his disc problems went away entirely. They only existed in the first place because he felt as though he was carrying the weight of the world on his shoulders.

I share this particular story because it illustrates how important it is to release pent-up feelings. It is not enough to "carry" powerful feelings and thoughts inside while you try to sort them out in the privacy of your own mind. That will keep you wrapped up in distorted logic and emotion, like a mouse running around in a maze. You must get your feelings and thoughts out. My client could not attain freedom from emotional and physical pain until he had a chance to release the emotional burden he was carrying.

In this chapter, I describe a number of techniques you can use by yourself to express your deeper emotions, release them, and make better sense of your *story behind the story*. These techniques are an essential and potent aid to healing when used in tandem with the other methods in this book. They'll be especially important to you if you don't have options for venting your powerful feelings and thoughts, which is unfortunately the case for many people. Perhaps you can no longer rely on your friends and family for emotional support; your problems have persisted for a long time and no one wants to listen to them anymore, so you clam up and feel cut off, as if there's a foot-thick wall of glass separating you from the rest of the world. Or perhaps your friends and family are deceased or have moved on, and you have no one to talk to. Or maybe you simply can't level with the other people in your life. If you fall into one or more of these categories, you can benefit immensely from the techniques in this chapter.

CATHARTIC RELEASE

Catharsis is the term used by modern psychology to describe the act of expressing deep emotions. You can use three effective cathartic release techniques to achieve freedom from pent-up emotion: venting your feelings aloud, writing or journaling your feelings, or working them out through exercise.

To vent your feelings aloud you only need two things: a set of working vocal chords and the ability to overcome a quirky social taboo. After all, only crazy people talk to themselves, right? Or maybe you believe it's all right to talk to yourself, as long as you don't talk back. Actually, it's OK to talk to yourself and equally OK to talk back. Human beings are expressive by nature. Just think of some of the technological and creative endeavors that have fueled the evolution of our society—the wheel, fine art, music, suspension bridges, the microprocessor, the space shuttle—none of which would be possible without expression. Verbal expression is natural and healthy to the species.

To vent your thoughts and feelings aloud, find some private time and simply speak the thoughts and feelings that are traveling through your mind. Tell it like it is, even if it's hurtful, distasteful, or even repugnant. What you think and feel will only find full release if you vent your thoughts and feelings *exactly* as they exist in your mind. If your feelings are powerful, feel free to put some "oomph" behind your oral expression. If you do it right, expect this technique to lead to possible tears, shouting, slamming your fist on the table, or other forms of physical release. Do whatever you need to do. That's the point of the exercise. If you're holding in emotional pain, take every opportunity to vent your feelings aloud until you find the release you need. You can use time spent on the road effectively in this way. You have complete anonymity when you're behind the wheel—just be sure to drive carefully as well.

The same rules hold for journaling or writing: to get the benefit of this technique you have to write *exactly* what you think and feel. Writing for cathartic release is not necessarily the same as expressive writing (EW) which I describe in the next section of this chapter. When you write for release, you want to write about your history (problems, losses, worries, fears, angers, betrayals, and so forth) just as they are. This is a "your-eyes-only" exercise, so you can afford to be honest and entirely truthful. If you try to make it "nice," it won't work.

Regular journaling is a therapeutic art. There are several styles of journaling and all have merit. Basic journaling is easy. Take a blank journal or notebook and start writing about how you feel right now. Describe your history and important relationships and the impact your past has had on who you are today. Be sure to chronicle the positive and the negative. Having explored your life story a bit, come back to the present. Then, at regular intervals (for some people, daily), chronicle the major events in your day and how you feel and think about them, along with how you behaved today and why. In doing so, you'll gain frequent release of otherwise difficult thoughts and feelings and be able to identify patterns—repetitive ways of relating to others and of feeling, thinking, and behaving in response to specific events or stresses in your environment. You'll be able to see with stark clarity just how much your past is influencing who you are today. This self-insight will give you another angle on your *story behind the story*.

Regular journaling is extremely therapeutic, but you can get the benefit of writing for cathartic release without it. Simply set aside some time and get out paper and pen. A computer will work, as well. Start by writing in a stream-of-consciousness fashion about the thing or things that are troubling you. Describe what has hurt you (illness, events, relationships) and the toll it's taken. Write down how you feel, any thoughts related to your feelings, or anything related to why you feel the way you do. You might ask yourself how you'd like to "fix" this problem or what you need in order to feel better. To get the benefit of this technique, I usually recommend a half hour of writing every day or every other day for about two weeks. You'll need that much time to address levels of thought and feeling that lie underneath the surface layers, as if you were peeling an onion.

If an important relationship has been a major source of pain in your life, you can choose to write a letter you never send to the person. Feel free to explore all your anger, frustration, fear, longing, or loss, or to demand restitution or express forgiveness, whatever applies. Just tell it like it is, and you'll get the release you're looking for. If the person you need to communicate with is no longer alive, or if your issues crosscut many years of strife, you can consider writing your letter to God or to the Universe.

If it's been a long time since you dealt authentically with your feelings you might need some "props" to help you engage your emotions more fully. Before you sit down to write for cathartic release, you could spend some time going through old photographs or mementos, or dig out some of your old music to listen to songs that had significance for you at a difficult time in your past. Such props are powerful triggers of memory and emotion.

Physical exercise is also a very potent means to cathartic release. Remember, your feelings and thoughts exist as subtle electromagnetic energy. When you exercise, you burn energy, including the harmful emotions and distorted thoughts that would otherwise sabotage your health and wellbeing. Many corporate CEOs and public school teachers, for example, effectively manage chronic mental stress with regular morning jogs, workouts at the gym, or frequent tennis. When I was in college, my roommate was a Golden Gloves bantamweight boxer, and he used to take me to the gym to work out twice a week. I was steeped in the social angst of the sixties in those days. I was determined to overcome all forms of social injustice and actively involved in the civil liberties movement. An hour in the ring twice a week gave me a release valve for the pressure and helped me keep things in perspective.

Exercise not only provides a means for cathartic release of emotion, it has the added benefits of improving physical health and increasing endorphin production, which boosts mental wellbeing. It also improves brain functioning by increasing blood and oxygen flow to the brain, helping to create new nerve cells and increasing chemicals in the brain that help cognition. Studies indicate that exercise is as effective in battling depression as anti-depressive medication.

You don't have to be a marathon runner to enjoy the cathartic benefits of physical exercise. Perhaps you are enduring chemotherapy or have orthopedic, neurological, viral, or other conditions that create major mobility and flexibility issues. If this is you, you'll need to exercise much less rigorously and should consult with your healthcare provider before embarking on any regimen. If your doctor tells you it's OK, consider walking or light bicycling, mild forms of yoga, flexibility exercises, or therapeutic stretching, all of which can suffice for cathartic release in folks with limited mobility and/or excessive bodily pain. You can also turn ordinary household chores into an exercise in cathartic release. I treated a woman many years ago who helped heal herself of severe arthritis by ritualizing ordinary housework. She imagined every cobweb or bathtub ring to be some aspect of her own frustration that she was "sweeping out." This woman lived with unrelenting levels of stress—a high powered job, a chronically ill child, financial difficulties from too much medical debt— but she arrested and reversed her arthritis through hypnosis, regular meditation, and "broom therapy."

EXPRESSIVE TECHNIQUES

A couple of years ago a middle-aged attorney came to me for help with depression, chronic fatigue, and frequent headaches. Her history was not terribly remarkable: raised in a loving family, she'd gone to law school with the dream of becoming an environmental advocate, but jobs in environmental law were hard to come by and she became a tax attorney instead. With the passage of time however, she found she hated her job. Her depression and fatigue grew and were now making it impossible for her to continue working.

Early on, I discovered this woman had an artistic temperament—she was a gifted painter and a pianist, though she hadn't applied these talents in years. On my encouragement, she started painting again and playing the piano. I suggested she do some expressive writing, and not long after, she found she had a gift for writing fiction. As she painted, played, and wrote, her depression cleared and the fatigue and headaches resolved. She is now in the process of getting her first book published and actively pursuing her dream to become a successful novelist.

This client's use of artistic expression was essential to her healing. Through painting, music, and writing, she was able to release her emotional pain, discover her creative nature, and become authentic to her *story behind the story*. She'd come from a middle-class family that strove hard for success. Her dad was a mid-level career bureaucrat who wanted the most for his daughter, and she'd gone to law school chiefly to please him. However, she was really an artist. For three decades of her adult life, *she didn't really know who she was*. She was living out her father's dream for her, a life that was inauthentic to her *story*. The result was depression, fatigue, and pain. Living a life that was consistent with her *story* brought her health and happiness.

The word "therapy" comes from the Greek word *therapeia*, which means to nurse or cure through creative expression—the arts, writing, music, dance, drama, gardening, hobbies, and creative play, just to name a few. You can use expressive techniques to attain cathartic release of old pain, symbolic resolution of issues that stand in the way of your complete healing, deeper self-knowledge, and joy.

With expressive techniques, the focus is on the change that comes to you through the process of creating. The focus is *not* on the aesthetics of the final product—you don't have to be a Michelangelo to get the benefit. I'm no artist, but I used painting to release my own deep emotions during my junior and senior years at college and my first year of graduate school. I would stretch out a huge canvas on the floor and toss large amounts of Rustoleum paint onto the canvas. I didn't use paintbrushes but I would sometimes swirl the paint splashes with a spatula or other objects. My approach (as I was to learn in later years) maximized what art therapists call "flow," a natural hypnotic state that focuses you entirely on a particular task. This is naturally restful and healing. My painting took an interesting turn during those years. It began with loud primary colors and harsh abrupt patterns—an expression of my angst in college—but I eventually found I preferred working with pastels and using fluid patterns—an expression of my maturation into peace and joy and my more sensual appreciation of what life has to offer.

As I did in this example, you might consider the arts (drawing, painting, photography, collage, mosaic work, sculpture, flower arranging, weaving, knitting, creative hobbies, and the like) as a means to access deep levels of self-expression. The language of the subconscious mind consists of symbols, metaphors, and deep feeling, so art provides a natural gateway for subconscious expression. Furthermore, time spent focusing on art will take your mind off what's stressing you. Just the act of having an artistic avocation can make you feel more balanced in life and provide you with more enjoyable downtime.

The benefits of artistic expression are numerous: inner conflict resolution, release of repressed emotion, enhanced self-awareness, a positive change in attitude, an increase in emotional wellbeing, and higher levels of inspiration, optimism, and personal growth. There are special benefits for people who suffer from physical illness. Studies show that artistic endeavors shift the body's physiology away from stress to one of deep relaxation by fostering different brain wave patterns, improving autonomic nervous system functioning and increasing the production of certain neurotransmitters in the brain. These changes boost immune system function and blood flow to vital organs. Studies with women also show that artistic expression improves hormone balance.

Creative writing is another very effective means for achieving emotional release, mental clarity, peace of mind, and improved health, especially for people who've experienced traumatic or otherwise stressful events in life. Creative writing has many forms. Expressive writing (EW) involves putting your thoughts and feelings down on paper, and you can use EW in a freeform way to address how you feel about your illness or important events and people in your life. You could also choose to write out your story as if you were a biographer looking at your life from the outside. One approach focuses on creating a dream-list—what you would do if you could do anything you wanted. Some people write expressively around the use of metaphors ("During this period in my life I feel like a butterfly in a chrysalis"). Regardless of how you approach it, EW is a process that brings release, clarity, and perspective to feelings, events, and directions in life that are otherwise chaotic or "unknowable." EW can take the form of writing only, or you can combine it with sketches, paintings, photographs, mementos, or art clipped from magazines. It is a particularly dynamic form of self-expression, and you can easily tailor it to your interests and personality type.

Poetry, in all its forms, provides a unique means of release and expression because of the special role that rhythm plays in writing—poetry tends to move the writer from one level of inspiration to another while expressing feelings at the same time. As with all of the other expressive techniques we're discussing here, you don't need to be a literary master to benefit from this. What you experience through the process is much more important than what you produce.

Fictional writing is an equally potent means for self-expression because of its mythic quality. The subconscious mind loves to communicate with stories—the more symbolic and metaphorical the better. With fiction, you can feel free to explore archetypal trends in your life, change your story, endow yourself (the hero in your story) with superhuman qualities, change your gender, height, or looks, or exaggerate the fiendish nature of the people or events that have plagued you. Far from being fantastic nonsense, this type of fictional exercise will help you make sense of your struggle and/or purpose in life, boost your self-esteem, and inspire you to live out your dreams.

You've probably heard of the "Mozart Effect," the power of certain types of music to drop physical and mental stress. Music—whether you listen to it or create it—has several benefits. Research suggests that music stimulates the body's natural "feel good" chemicals (opiates and endorphins) and subtly improves blood pressure, pulse rate, breathing, immune system functioning, and posture. Music as sound therapy has been used to treat stress, grief, depression, schizophrenia, and autism in children, as well as diagnose mental health needs. The nice thing about music is you can access it around the clock—in the car, via your IPod on the walk to work, or on the home stereo. You may prefer to kick back in reverie to the soaring strains of Vivaldi or blast southern rock while you're in the kitchen making dinner. With music, it's different strokes for different folks. Just watch out for harsh discordant sounds—this type of music is good for release of powerful emotion, but a steady diet of it will drive too much negative energy into your subconscious mind and BioEM field.

I have trouble listening to music without dancing. I may not be Fred Astaire, but I like to cut a rug now and then because it makes me feel good. Dance is therapeutic because of the vital connection between movement and the emotional, intellectual, and physical energies that make up your BioEM field. Dance or movement can therefore help integrate and harmonize the emotional, physical, and cognitive facets of "self." Movement provides a kinesthetic pathway for subconscious memories, conflicts, and issues to express and release (in much the same way exercise does). Those recovering from physical, sexual, or emotional abuse may find this expressive technique especially helpful for gaining a sense of ease with their own bodies.

Not everyone is ballroom material of course—some of us feel like we have two left feet, but there are still options for gaining the benefit of dance or movement as a form of expressive release. When nobody's watching, put on some music and give yourself permission to move in whatever way you feel like moving. You can experience movement as tension release, dwell on a particular situation, thought, or emotion as you're dancing, or you can simply move with the music. The amount of emotional release you enjoy might surprise you. Symbols, metaphors, or old memories might crop up as you continue to move. You might feel like shedding a tear, you might begin to feel downright joyful, or both. For those of you who need a structured setting in order to "move" you might consider a dance class, dance therapy, attending a local ballroom dance, or even taking a class in Tai Chi, aikido, or yoga.

Aristotle first mentioned the word *catharsis* to describe emotional release in audiences who were watching tragic Greek plays. Dramatic expression—whether you watch it or do it—refers to the use of theater to facilitate emotional release, personal growth, and improved health. You can use expression through drama to achieve catharsis, solve a problem, delve deeply into truths about yourself, understand the meaning of personally resonant images, or transcend unhealthy patterns of interaction. There are formal "drama therapies" used in settings like hospitals, schools, mental health centers, and businesses. Here, therapeutic drama includes psychodrama, role-play, theater games, group-dynamic games, mime, puppetry, and improvisational techniques—even stand-up comedy.

If you would like to explore drama as a means of self-expression, you can turn to any number of drama, madrigal, or theater groups in your local community, but as Aristotle said, you can also get the benefits of dramatic expression just by attending a good play, ballet, opera, or movie. Audience members get deeply involved in the plot of a good performance and connect in a mythic, archetypal way with the struggles and triumphs of the main characters. There's a reason why movies like the *Lord of the Rings* trilogy are so popular. Many people resonate with Eowyn (the princess warrior archetype), Frodo (the humble savior archetype), or Gandalf (the wise sage).

You can also weave a little dramatic expression into your day-to-day living by experimenting with role-play, comedy, and improvisation. You know the old adage, "More truth was said in jest than ever was said in sorrow." In the late evenings, my family members often gather in the kitchen. If one of us has had a hard day, that person will often "act out" his or her dilemma with tremendous theatrical or comic exaggeration, while the rest of us join in the show. An ordinary exercise in "kitchen drama" like this can achieve a great deal of cathartic release, healing, and understanding.

You can gain the benefits of expressive release through any creative endeavor, from building models to gardening to cooking a gourmet meal. Working with your hands to create something is cathartic, restful to the mind and body, and *grounding*; it connects you into the here and now and helps alleviate stress. Feelings of appreciation, tranquility, and joy tend to accompany a creative act, especially if you are concentrating fully on your enterprise (which invites a natural hypnotic state). Gardening is particularly good for this because it combines elements of exercise and creativity in a healthful outdoor setting. Studies indicate that it produces substantial benefits to physical and mental health for people of all ages. It reduces blood pressure, alleviates negative emotions and stressful thoughts, boosts mood and brain functioning, and improves motivation and morale.

USE OF THESE TECHNIQUES

I suggest you consider the techniques in this chapter, determine which methods feel right to you, and begin experimenting with them now. These techniques rarely stand alone as a cure for physical illness, but they are powerful adjuncts to your plan for attaining miraculous health. In the next chapter, I will help you figure out how to integrate these techniques with the other methods in this book as part of your personalized plan for success.

PART FIVE

PREPARING FOR THE REST OF YOUR LIFE

CHAPTER 15

WHERE TO GO FROM HERE

I n writing this book, I was determined to give you everything you need to accomplish your goals for miraculous health. In the preceding chapters, I provided you with the same level of information I usually deliver to my clients over six months of visits to my office. You've just had a crash course in the latest techniques of mind-body medicine. In this chapter, I'll show you how to bring it all together to structure a plan for achieving your goals and then help you set the tone for a lifetime of health and ultimate wellbeing.

By now, you realize that, although you came to this book because you had concerns about your physical health, healing is about more than "fixing" those problems. It's about being authentic to your *story behind the story*. What's been going on in your body has been the result of psychological, spiritual, and physical interactions and the unintended consequence of not realizing how deep and powerful your mind is.

The road to miraculous health is self-empowering. You're about to become a major player in your own healthcare. There is a general rule of thumb that's applied by advanced practitioners of mind-body medicine: if you suffer from a physical illness or injury, about 40 percent of your solution will come from physical means (such as surgery, medication, physical therapy, changes in diet, and increased exercise), and the other 60 percent will come from your mind. You now have the tools you need to activate that other 60 percent of your healthcare solution. In fact, your mind is so powerful that you have the ability to compensate for situations where traditional medicine doesn't deliver on its end of the bargain. You will never again passively receive healthcare, nor will you rely only on your healthcare providers to give you everything you need to sustain your health. From now on, you're in charge.

What to Expect

People often ask me, "Why do some get a sensational benefit from the methods while others have to work with their tools for a while?" Three factors will determine how quickly you will heal from the use of these methods:

- The severity of your problem
- The degree to which you are authentically engaging your *story behind the story*
- The degree to which you maintain a receptive attitude

Long-term chronic illness can take more time to heal. Many years ago, I had the privilege of treating a young man who suffered from disabling rheumatoid arthritis. He was a South American diplomat who, though only in his late thirties, could hardly move his fingers. All his joints were stiff and inflamed, and he lived in constant severe pain. A man of some means, he'd been to several doctors and tried many traditional and alternative treatments for his problem—even experimental gold injections. Nothing helped.

This man endured a very stressful early life due to high levels of political upheaval in his home country. I started doing regular energy healing work on him, introduced him to meditation, and used hypnotic regression to help him release old trauma. His health improvements came slowly (though measurably), but he maintained an optimistic attitude throughout. He stuck with his program for two years and even extended his diplomatic stay in the United States so he could complete his work with me. During this period, the amount of time between our sessions lengthened, based on how long he could go without experiencing pain. Eventually, the pain went away completely.

Stress and arthritis are closely related. When we finished our work together, this man returned to his country and resumed his primary responsibility: attempting to eradicate his homeland from drug-traffickers. In this job, his life was on the line daily. He kept in touch with me for five years after he returned to South America, and despite the inordinate stress, his arthritis did not return.

This was a particularly long-term and severe case, but it underscores a point: stick with your plan until it delivers. Everyone wants the "big hit," and as I've demonstrated through the case histories in this book, many people get it. However, if that is not you, keep going. You will certainly enjoy noticeable incremental improvements in your health. Just work with your tools until they deliver everything you need from them.

The second factor has to do with how well you're working with your *story behind the story*. If you are moving in tandem with it, you will make rapid progress. If you resist your lessons, you'll find your progress to be slow and incremental. What's happening here is that your subconscious mind is purposely slowing your progress in an effort to get you to connect with your *story behind the story*. If your progress is very slow, you're not seeing or acknowledging something, and your subconscious mind won't let you make significant progress until you do so.

I am now working with a very prominent man to help him overcome stomach cancer. This man has worked with U.S. presidents, formed a powerful think tank, and sits on the boards of many beneficent organizations. By anyone's account, he is highly successful and has helped millions of people. We began our work by using a wide range of techniques, including hypnotic regression and meditation, the Gearshift, and energy healing work. Despite his stature in the world, this man found himself plagued by self-doubt. His father, the mayor of the city in California where he grew up, was overly harsh and critical toward him. As a result, my client became driven, always trying to prove himself in the world.

As he began to employ the methods, he started to shift away from being a "big-shot" and toward a simpler way of being. Deepening experience in meditation led him to return to his Catholic roots, and he started going to mass every day. He felt he wanted to come to know God and work more directly for human welfare. He went to work as the head of one of the world's largest humanitarian aid organizations. As he continued to deepen his spirituality, he shifted his focus even further. He volunteered in one of the organizations that he oversaw as a board member, and for six months he worked with a poor, uneducated man and taught him to read. Only then did he find a modicum of the peace he was looking for.

But his story doesn't end there. Despite his personal growth, this man still hasn't fully let go of worldly power as a marker of success because he hasn't gained perfect freedom from self-doubt. Since this is the case, he still has significant physical problems to contend with. He's doing good work, though, a determined man of great heart who should prevail over his cancer as he continues to live more authentically with his story.

This man is still in treatment with me. I purposely didn't pick a "happily ever after" story in this case because going deeply into your *story behind the story* can surprise you. It may not fit your preexisting values or the world's idea of success. In this instance, my client's *story* called him away from being a major mover and shaker to the depths of spiritual humility. That would be an extremely tough transition for most people, and it has not been entirely easy for him. Remember, though, that it's not how big you are that counts; it's how real you are and how authentic you're being to your highest aspirations. Finding and living out your *story* is the purpose of life. You've come to this book because you or someone you love has significant health issues. This book will help you overcome those. In addition, it will take you to your higher goal—to strive hard to live out your noblest destiny, as best you can perceive it, no matter where it leads you. Your overall health depends on it.

The third factor that will have an impact on how quickly you make progress is your level of receptivity toward the methods and science behind them. These methods are powerful and the science that backs them is solid. They are like a seed that carries the potential to become the most majestic tree in the forest; but there is the power of the seed, and then there's the receptivity of the soil. How receptive are you to the power of these methods and to your own power? The monthly publication of the National Guild of Hypnotists recently featured an article by a well-trained hypnotherapist who decided to do a little experiment with himself. He had a heart problem for which he took medication and decided to use his hypnotic skills to heal his heart. This man traveled extensively and shortly after starting his experiment, he had to go on a lengthy road trip. He threw his heart medication in his travel bag. During a month on the road, he continued to do hypnotic work on his heart and was able to cut his heart medication in half with no negative health effects. He arrived back home feeling smug about his success. Only when he unpacked did he realize he'd put the wrong medication in his luggage. For the length of his trip, he'd been taking a cold pill instead of his heart medication. He'd healed his heart, but his expectation was that he was reliant on meds to begin with and that he'd have to reduce this dependency slowly. The joke was on him. If fate hadn't intervened, who knows how long it would've taken him to heal his heart. As you move forward to undertake this journey, do it without limits on your expectations and a truly open mind. It will make an enormous difference.

Your Plan for Attaining Miraculous Health

Before you start on your treatment plan, you should quickly review your starting baseline and take stock of where you are now. This baseline will consist chiefly of the self-rating scales you used in chapter 5, along with any objective medical data you have at your disposal (such as your blood sugar, blood pressure and cholesterol levels, recent X-rays or scans, lab work results, or physician reports). Now you're ready to go.

Structuring a plan that will let you achieve your goals is actually simple. We're going to approach it as if you were dining out at your local restaurant, where there's both a fixed and an à la carte menu. First, let's review all the items on the menu—the tools you now have at your disposal:

- Alpha-III Download—Hypnotic Meditation (Meditate on your own without the hypnotic assist if you prefer.)
- Gamma-I Download—The Stressbuster
- Gamma-II Download—Hypnotic Imagery to Target Illness in the Body
- Gamma-III Download—Hypnotic Pain Relief
- Gamma-IV Download—Hypnotic Weight Loss
- Gamma-V Download—Hypnotic Regression
- Gamma-VI Download—Hypnotic Energy Healing
- Gamma-VII Download—The Gearshift Exercise

- Cognitive Reprogramming
- Expressive Techniques

For the first three weeks, I recommend you try the following selections from the menu, with the indicated frequency:

Phase one fixed menu:
- Hypnotic Meditation three times per week
- Hypnotic Regression once a week
- The Stressbuster two times per week
- Hypnotic Energy Healing once a week

I designed this fixed menu to cut your stress immediately, activate the body's immune system, expand your awareness, relieve anxiety and depression, grant you freedom from old emotional pain, and deliver increased levels of energy to your body to jump-start the healing process. Try alternating meditation with the other methods, so that you are meditating approximately every other day and using one of the other methods in between.

If you suffer from severe pain or if weight gain is complicating your health status, you will want to do the following exercises in *addition* to the above:

Phase one à la carte menu:
- Hypnotic Pain Relief every other day
- Hypnotic Weight Loss every other day

After you've followed this menu for three weeks, take stock of your health and wellbeing. Go back to the self-rating scales and reevaluate your status. Note the changes and any progress you've made. If you can assess relevant objective health indicators, such as resting heart rate, blood pressure, or blood sugar levels, do this and jot down the readings. Then, make a few notes about any other material differences in how you think or feel emotionally and physically. These would be things like, "I feel less angry and more optimistic," or "I have more energy." Record negative observations, as well, "I feel more sadness." If this is you, it just means you're making progress because you are getting in touch with repressed feelings that have been sabotaging your health. Continued application of the methods will free you from negative thoughts and feelings, but first you have to get them up and out. This is a sign of growth, not a sign that there's a problem.

Now you're ready to move forward. For the next three weeks, try the following selections from the menu:

Phase two fixed menu:
- Hypnotic Meditation three times per week
- The Stressbuster once a week
- Hypnotic Energy Healing once a week
- The Gearshift Exercise once a week
- Hypnotic Imagery to target illness in the body once a week

This fixed menu will continue delivering the essential benefits of the phase one strategy (stress reduction, increased immune functioning, freedom from depression and anxiety, and increased energy flow). However, we've added two methods that will allow you to go after the illness or injury in your body more aggressively: the Gearshift and Hypnotic Imagery. We've taken Hypnotic Regression off the fixed menu at this point because you will already have enjoyed substantial emotional release through its use during phase one. You will return to it later on an as-needed basis. Remember to alternate meditation with the other methods so that you are meditating approximately every other day.

If you suffer from chronic pain or have a problem with excessive weight, you will want to continue doing the following exercises *in addition* to the above:

Phase two à la carte menu:
- Hypnotic Pain Relief every other day
- Hypnotic Weight Loss every other day

Once you've followed this new menu for three weeks, you'll want to reevaluate your status in precisely the same way you did before. Chart your progress. At this point, it should be considerable when compared to your starting baseline of six weeks ago.

From this point on, design your own program. Rely on hypnotic meditation three days per week and fill-in the remaining four days with the methods that best fit your needs and learning style. You are smart enough to be your own guide and by this time will have gained enough familiarity with the methods to know what seems to be working for you. It is probably a good idea to keep the Gearshift Exercise in your weekly regimen because of its power. Use it first to focus on healing your body and then move on to goals that are most essential to fulfilling your *story behind the story.* If you feel as though you need more emotional release, put Hypnotic Regression back on the menu for a while until you find the release you need. You can also begin experimenting with Expressive Techniques. If you are still dealing with too much pain, stay with Hypnotic Pain Relief until you get results. Everyone can benefit from using the Cognitive Reprogramming method, especially those of you who "think a lot." You can use this method often, twenty-four hours a day, seven days a week, to improve the gains you're making with your daily hypnotic or meditative practice.

Whatever you decide to do, stay with your new plan for three weeks, then evaluate your progress. If it appears to be working, stay with the same strategy for another three weeks. Feel free to shift the strategy at three-week intervals in whatever way feels right. Your needs will change over time, and you'll want to experiment with different ways of packaging the methods. Remember that the methods gain in power as you continue to use them, so stick with any particular menu for three weeks. The exception exists in a case where you find a method too difficult, as might be the case if you experience too much emotional release when you're doing Hypnotic Regression work. If this happens, stop using this method and consult a mental healthcare professional before you proceed any further with it.

The pace I've outlined—employing at least one method every day—is ideal. However, you might find that it is too rapid for you, either because you cannot handle this much change this rapidly or because you simply don't have the time to employ the methods every day (perhaps you are nursing a chronically ill child around the clock or work in a profession that requires you to be on call for multiple shifts). It's fine to slow things down a little bit, as long as you keep at it. Try to meditate twice per week and add two of the other methods into the days between. You'll make progress this way, even if that progress isn't as fast. If the opportunity arises to get to the ideal of daily use, take it.

MIRACULOUS HEALTH IS ONLY THE BEGINNING

You've now had a glimpse of your greatness. You understand that in order to heal your body you will have to engage your *story behind the story* with the utmost sincerity and depth—and you have the tools to do that. Very soon, you will achieve your goals for improved health.

Then what?

You will have become powerful enough to stay with your current story or rewrite your story altogether. The decision is entirely yours.

Essentially, two kinds of people come to see me. The first want to maintain their lives with a few adjustments. Maybe they want better physical or mental health, a better marriage, a higher income, more time to travel, or more leisure. For these folks, the purpose of life is to go with the flow and enjoy the simple pleasures, such as love of family and friends.

The second group is composed of the adventurers. They love to blow the lid off the status quo. They want to know what comes next and they want to go for it. They're interested in reinventing their story. They don't care much about the cultural stereotypes of the "good life."

Why can't you do both? You don't have to be caught in the "Alexander dichotomy," opting for a short glorious life and an early demise like Alexander the Great. Nor do you have to settle for a conventional ripe old age of measured progress. Using the methods in this book, you can easily unleash enough mental power to do both and live a long life of no limits.

What do you want most out of life? Surprisingly few people ever ask themselves that question. You've had to answer it as you worked through the process in this book because the answer is integral to your *story behind the story* and to your health. You can use the methods in this book to expand your awareness. If you do, your *story* will continue to unfold and an endless stream of possibilities will open up. Your potential is limitless because your mind is *infinite*; it is the highest purpose of life to discover this truth. Health, wealth, power, possessions—even a great love in your life—all take a backseat to the *ultimate story behind your story*, which is to discover just how powerful you really are.

Welcome to your new life. You're going to love living it.

BONUS CHAPTER

SEEING THINGS IN A NEW WAY

My guess is that now that you've discovered the remarkable power available to you when you unleash your mind, you're not quite ready to stop. If that's the case, you might enjoy the "bonus" I've prepared for you: one last mental skill that can enhance your life. Let's start with a quick exercise that will offer you a chance to explore the potential of acquiring vision skills—the ability to see electromagnetic energies.

It's good to wait to do this one until you go to sleep at night, as this works better when it's dark. If you decide to do this in the daytime, pull the curtains and make the room as dark as possible. Then lie down and relax, but leave your eyes open.

For a few moments, focus on your breath as it moves in and out of your body. Then count yourself down from ten to one. Remember to do this slowly, allowing about three seconds between numbers.

When you've counted down, let your gaze go a little bit by purposely not focusing on any one object in the room. Imagine a spot halfway between you and the ceiling or between you and the opposite wall, and let your eyes fall on that area without trying to focus explicitly on anything in particular. For the next two minutes, imagine that you are starting to fall asleep. Let your eyes relax and your vision becomes slightly diffuse and unfocused. You just want to space out.

As you do this, you'll start to notice the darkness in the room isn't uniform anymore. You'll see it has texture. Some parts seem a little darker, others lighter, while some parts seem dense and others diaphanous—like a silk veil you can see through. You begin to perceive little clouds or pockets of variation in density. You will observe that, if you focus too narrowly on any one cloud, it might disappear, so keep your gaze relaxed and unfocused.

Now let yourself relax even more. You might notice little specks of light that "flash" in the darkness, like the white spots on one of those old-fashioned composition notebooks but smaller. Do you see these coming and going?

You are starting to see electromagnetic energies. You have been seeing them all your life and probably didn't pay any attention to them. Perhaps you dismissed them as a smear on your eyeglasses or chalked them up to eyestrain. However, they are real. In this chapter, I will show you how to see them more clearly and understand what they mean.

Many years ago, it was my practice to do Social Security disability evaluations on a low-rate basis for the state of Maryland. One case involved a man who arrived at my office on the arm of his wife. He'd had a severe stroke two years prior. In his mid fifties, Mexican by birth, he headed a mid-sized corporation of about 200 employees at the time of his stroke. Now, he could hardly talk. Stuttering, almost unintelligible, he began to speak haltingly of his pain, "I . . . It . . . i-is . . . hard. . . ."

The family was Catholic and devout. During the evaluation, I learned that a priest from their archdiocese, who was a gifted healer, had been working regularly with the man. The priest even had a room in their house where he would stay over, but he hadn't been able to help.

When I finished the evaluation, I offered to do some energy work on the man. I hoped he would be open to it, based on his openness to healing from the priest. In fact, he was eager to try. I asked him to stand. Using my vision skills (my ability to see electromagnetic energies), I had already scanned his BioEM energy field while I was conducting his evaluation. His energy field was dampened around his head (meaning there was too little energy flow), and there was a lot of gray (the color of physical illness) and red (the color of physical pain) concentrated in the area of his brain dysfunction.

As I began doing biofield energy work on his head, I could see green energy (the color of healing) flowing from my hand into the energy field around his head. At first, the energy from my hand would dissipate the gray and red, replacing these colors with green and a little gold (which indicates peace). If I stopped for even a moment, though, the gray and red came back. I kept working, super-loading my patient's energy field with healing energy until finally his entire field shifted from gray and red to gold.

He was trying to speak as I worked on him—an excruciatingly slow, halted effort to tell me about his guilt regarding his wife. Just as his energy field shifted entirely to gold, he shifted into lucid speech. He moved from stumbling over a disjointed stream of words that went something like, "I . . . f-f-feel . . . bad . . . w-w-wife . . . alone," into a fluid, articulate statement, ". . . and I feel so guilty because I can't be there for her." Then he startled and shouted, "Oh my God, Oh, my God, Oh, my God, I'm back," and the three of us cried in each other's arms.

EVERYONE CAN SEE BioEM ENERGIES

Human beings have the natural ability to see BioEM energies. Children see them often and easily, right up until their cultural conditioning (family life, academic work, social pressure, and so on) forces them to focus on their environment in a different way. We tend not to "see" energy because we're trained to focus pointedly on discrete objects, not on the space around them. In my work with indigenous cultures where the norm is not to focus on a specific object but on a larger field of vision, it is typical and understandable for people to see energy.

I've been teaching people to see BioEM energies for nearly two decades and about 90 percent of participants are able to see "something" of the BioEM field, with 70 percent being able to see specific colors and patterns with substantial detail and accuracy after just one seminar.

THE VALUE OF READING BioEM ENERGY FIELDS

Dr. Harold Saxton Burr did the most interesting work on electromagnetic fields at Yale Medical School in the teens through the 1950s. Burr wrote a book called *Blueprint for Immortality* that explained how you could detect all kinds of physical problems in the energy field before you could identify them through traditional diagnosis. Doing so has a huge impact on many healthcare problems where time is of the essence, such as cancer. I've used this "early diagnostic method" myself many times, where simply by looking at someone's energy field, I can identify cancer in that person before there is anything manifest in the body. With a jump like that, we can knock the cancer out quickly before it has a chance to do real damage.

By reading someone's BioEM field, you receive a lot of detailed information—not just about what's happening in the body but about the personality, what that person is thinking, what that person feels at the time, how he or she operates, and so forth. In other words, you will be able to "see" physical disease in the body, along with important diagnostic information related to its mental and spiritual root causes. I will show you how to do this before the close of this chapter.

In chapter 2 we discussed *feeling* BioEM energy. The visioning skills in this chapter will allow you to *see* it. The two are essentially a check on each other. Some people are better at seeing energy than they are at feeling or "sensing" it, and vice versa. You should try to develop both. They are complimentary, and if you develop your visioning skills, you will receive added diagnostic information.

THE METHOD

Before you start, download Alpha-III from www.miraculoushealthbook.com, burn it to a CD, and set up the room the way you have elsewhere in this book. All the instruction you'll need to gain the experience of seeing BioEM energy is included in the download, but let me prep you a little.

To do this exercise you need a "subject," a human being to observe. The best way to do it is with a partner. If you don't have a partner to work with, you can be your own subject with the use of a body-length mirror. In either case, have the person you're going to read (either your partner or yourself) stand up about an inch or two away from a white wall in a room with indirect, slightly dimmed incandescent lighting. Later, you'll be able to read people in any setting, but for now, try to employ these ideal conditions—they'll help you see the energies more clearly.

Ask the person you are going to read to stand still and make sure there are no shadows being cast anywhere near that person.

Now place your gaze loosely on the chest and neck of the person you are reading. You're not trying to focus intently on the person. You can't drive this experience; you just need to relax enough to let it come to you.

While your eyes are fixed loosely on your subject, focus your mind on the periphery of the body—at first the upper half of the body, parts of the arms, the shoulders, the neck, around the head, then outward in the air immediately surrounding the upper body

Now start the download. In it, you'll hear me do a ten-to-one countdown like the one we used in the hypnosis exercises. You'll follow the lulling tone of my voice and drift even further into a passive-receptive laid-back attitude while continuing to look at your subject and the air around the body in a diffuse, unfocused way.

Simply follow the remaining instructions on the download and observe what you notice along the way. At this point, most people start to see an outline around the body of the person they're reading. What you see will vary depending on your subject's energy field and on how deeply you allow yourself to move with the exercise. Most people will see a gray, silver, yellow, or silvery-white outline that is one-quarter inch to two inches wide. If the line you see is gray, you might think it is a shadow, but you'll soon realize that it doesn't really look like a shadow at all. What you're seeing is the "etheric" BioEM field, which is copying the shape of the body. The colors—gray, silver, or yellow—do not carry special diagnostic significance. Occasionally though, other colors will bleed into this field if the person you are reading has some level of weakness, particularly if that person is under chronic stress.

Out beyond the etheric BioEM field is another part of the field called the astral BioEM field (*astral* means light). This part of the field extends several feet out in all directions from the body in an ovular shape. Its energies are associated with the physical, psychological, and spiritual aspects of a person. The astral field may exhibit a spectrum of colors, different shapes, and motion, all of which have important diagnostic significance. You may not be able to see the astral BioEM field immediately, but if you practice this visioning technique a few times, you should be able to see at least a few colors and some movement right away. With continued practice, you will be able to see the astral field in great detail.

To deepen the experience, play the instruction download again. At this point, there's an excellent chance you'll begin to see pale colors in the astral field, maybe a little purple or some red with little clouds of bright yellow and waves of color flowing out from the body. This is your first step toward using vision skills for diagnosis. If you want to have some fun, do this exercise a few times with a couple of friends, and enjoy comparing notes as you *all* come to see precisely the same play of color and light while looking at another person's BioEM field.

WHAT THE COLORS MEAN

Colors in the astral BioEM field provide important diagnostic information regarding a person's physical, mental, and spiritual health:

Once you build your skill of seeing the colors in the astral BioEM field, you will begin to notice variations in location, shape, and motion in the field. These also have something unique to reveal about a person.

COLOR	DEFINITION/MEANING
GOLD	Represents the deepest levels of peace. Very deep gold represents spiritual peace.
WHITE	Indicates purity. It can mean spiritual purity, though some people are extremely pure (virtuous, loving, and kind) and have never even heard of God.
PURPLE	Represents a service nature, the kind of people devoted to community service or cleaning up the kitchen after a meal.
RED	Signifies intensity of emotion. Most often indicates anger and/or fear but can represent positive emotion. Also indicates physical pain when localized tightly around a body part.
GRAY	Reflects a number of different conditions, most frequently sadness and depression, where it is often seen in combination with red because repressed anger and fear create depression. Gray is present when people are very tired, physically ill (or about to become so), taking medication, or using drugs and/or alcohol. Gray shimmering with sparkly light signifies anxiety and worry. If you see gray in someone's field, you'll need to ask some questions to get the right interpretation.

Color	Definition/Meaning
GREEN	The color of healing. People who are healing well have green in their field. A lot of green indicates that the person is moving more healing energy than needed and would make a good healer. Green can also signify creativity.
PINK	Signifies good health. A healthy person is literally "in the pink."
ORANGE	Indicates a healthy self-esteem. As this color deepens, it signifies humility.
BLUE	Represents thought. Dark blue tends to indicate worldly thinking. Robin's egg blue tends to indicate spiritual thinking.
AQUA	As a combination of blue and green, aqua represents healing qualities within a thought-oriented individual. It is usually dark and intense, a particularly striking color in the field.
YELLOW	An indication of intellectual defense mechanisms. Some yellow is healthy because it shows the person's ability to stay on track. A great deal of yellow indicates that a person is blocking too much. Eventually, such a person ends up with gray in their fields, the color of depression.
BROWN	Signifies self-doubt. People with a lot of brown in their fields tend to have real issues with self-esteem, self-identity, and what they stand for in life. They tend to be extremely hard on themselves, almost to the point where they're digging into themselves emotionally.
BLACK	Very rarely seen in the BioEM field, black indicates the presence of the severest emotional/spiritual problems. It usually signifies the presence of evil.

Location of color will provide insight. For example, if you look at the field around a person's head, you can learn a great deal about his or her personality. If you see colors very close to the body, the person is likely to be consciously *aware* of the issues associated with those colors, whereas colors farther away from the body indicate feelings or traits that are in the person's subconscious mind (which means he or she is probably unaware of them). The dividing line appears to be between nine and fifteen inches from the physical body and will vary depending on how strong the person's energy field is (the stronger the field, the farther out this dividing line lies).

Often, colors will appear in the astral BioEM field in the form of specific shapes. A circle full of color indicates the issue corresponding to the color has power in the person's life. Multi-sided figures (triangles, squares, pentagons) indicate that the issue has taken on significant power for the person, and the person is holding it with too much stress. Depending on the color (red, for example), there is some potential for explosion regarding these issues.

Motion in the astral field also has significant meaning. As you observed in the table, a uniform gray usually indicates sadness, depression, and physical illness, but a gray that is shimmering with activity indicates anxiety. As your visioning skills improve, you will notice swirling motions of layered energy moving in and around a particular area of a person's body. This motion usually reflects how reactive versus how centered and calm the individual may be, especially as correlated with issues that are symbolically or historically located in that part of the body. For example, a lot of swirling motion around the heart would indicate intense reactive feelings going on regarding loved ones and family.

OUR FIELDS INTERACT

As we've discussed earlier, we are all connected energetically. This fact becomes dramatically clear once you learn to see BioEM fields.

A few years ago, I was teaching a class for psychologists and psychiatrists. One of the female psychologists in attendance walked in on the first day of the class and sat next to one of the male psychologists. I noticed that, while their bodies were straight in their chairs, their energy fields leaned into one another. It was obvious to me that they had a personal relationship. The colors they had in common ran together like a river, even if the colors came from different parts of their bodies. This told me they knew one another extremely well and had a strong level of intuitive communication.

They kept their relationship quiet at first, but eventually they told everyone that they lived together and one of the reasons they took the class was to learn more about the intense spiritual connection they shared with each other. A year and a half later, I attended their marriage in West Virginia.

Of course, the way our energy fields interact isn't always so benign. As you come to use these skills, you'll notice there are people who cannibalize other people's energy fields. I've seen this in the workplace on numerous occasions. Someone will be sitting down minding his own business, doing his work. In comes the office jerk, a person who is hostile, with a big chip on his shoulder. He walks into the other person's cubicle and starts talking with a critical edge in his voice. If you read his energy field, you'll notice a sudden thrust—like an arrow—coming out from his field and invading his "victim's" field to "bite" a chunk of the other's energy. He steals his coworker's energy and leaves the victim feeling drained and anxious.

Another more common example is the energy-drained friend who calls you on the phone to complain about life. You try to offer some good advice, but this person discounts what you have to say or blows it off. Have you ever had a conversation like this where you feel completely spent afterward? If you'd watched the exchange using your vision skills, you would actually have seen the energy being drawn out of you by the erstwhile energy-hungry friend. The distance between callers doesn't matter.

ENERGY FIELDS AND THE HEALING PROCESS

As you continue to practice this technique, you'll start seeing the colors with greater accuracy, farther and farther from the body. Knowing what you now know about what color, location, shape, and motion mean in the BioEM field, you'll be able to use your vision skills to help identify maladies in yourself and others. You will actually be able to see the things that cause illness and contribute to illness. For example, you may notice someone you know is carrying a great deal of pain because you can see intense red flaring out from her right shoulder. You use your vision skills to gain a better picture of the *entire* malady: you see the gray of despair and sadness (which is making the pain even worse), some purple (your friend is very service-oriented; she volunteers at the local homeless shelter), some white around her head (she's a pure-hearted sweetie), and some brown (she suffers from self-doubt). You'll realize your friend is shouldering the burdens of others at her own expense, sacrificing too much of herself and probably thinking she's not good enough in the process.

Once you've become adept at the skills you've been learning in this book, you'll know what to do to help yourself and others. You can become quite the expert diagnostician by practicing your visioning skills. However, interpreting what you see and knowing how to treat it will require some additional knowledge and a huge dose of compassion. In this simple example, you might give your friend the name and number of a good orthopedist or physical therapist, but you would also invite her out for lunch and a pedicure, boost her self-esteem, and venture to ask her why she insists on making so many sacrifices for others at her own expense. Her answer would indicate what you should do next. Perhaps when she was a little girl, her parents were emotionally distant and she learned to sacrifice her essential needs in order to get the attention she desperately wanted.

Sometimes what you see in a person's energy field and what they should *do* about it aren't obvious. For example, let's say you read a person's BioEM field, and it's chock-full of red energy, signifying extreme anger. There's a lot of yellow in the field, signaling strong intellectual defenses, and a lot of shimmering gray, the color of anxiety. Is this person in trouble? Perhaps, but it depends. You'd have to know more about his history. The amount of red in his field could be a sign that he's emoting more, letting that old anger go, which is precisely what he should be doing in order to heal. It may not be pleasant for those around him, but it's healthy and understandable. If you were the friend of such a person, you might congratulate him and let him know you're available if he feels a need to vent his feelings. You would be a good friend by lending a sympathetic ear.

A good therapist knows how to find the root mental cause behind people's distorted thoughts, feelings, and actions and knows precisely how to lead them into freedom. As you do the work I've introduced you to in this book, you'll become a good therapist to yourself and to those you love.

YOUR TEN-DAY PLAN FOR DEVELOPING VISION SKILLS

There is nothing complicated about this process, but you will definitely get more out of it with practice. Set up the conditions described earlier in this chapter and try to work on your vision skills every day for ten days. As you do, you'll start seeing more and more.

After the first ten days of practice under ideal conditions, you'll be able to practice seeing BioEM energies anywhere and anytime. Look for ways to practice—in a restaurant, on the street, at the office. Just don't go around staring at strangers.

Eventually, you'll get so good at seeing BioEM energies and have so much information about people, that you'll learn to turn it off to avoid being impolite.

NOW YOU'RE READY FOR A LIFE WITHOUT LIMITS

Over three decades of clinical work, I have demonstrated that the power of the human mind is infinite, every person possesses extraordinary nobility, and life is a series of lessons designed to lead us into the direct experience of these truths. Using your ability to see bio-electromagnetic energies, together with the other tools in this book, you will come to experience this reality and live out your future in epic fashion—with no limits—in whatever way has the most meaning to you.

GLOSSARY

Archetype—Basic personality patterns that are lived out individually and from deep inside the collective culture. The accepted use of archetype refers to a generic or defining example of a personality type, such as a warrior, caregiver, or teacher. In the analysis of personality, archetype is often broadly used to refer to a stereotype, especially an oversimplification or epitome of type, such as the "greatest" warrior, caregiver, or teacher. These archetypal patterns run deep and can be accessed using hypnotic work, meditation, or psychotherapy to promote healing and self-understanding.

Authoritarian hypnosis—Hypnosis that emphasizes mind control methods, where the hypnotist is viewed as having special mental powers which cause the subject (person being hypnotized) to become vulnerable to the suggestions of the hypnotist. A well-known example of authoritarian hypnosis is stage hypnosis. Mind control methods do not take into account the free will of the subject and are rarely used in present-day clinical settings.

Belief system—A person's philosophical framework for receiving, generating, and sustaining knowledge. An individual's belief system is highly subjective and dependent upon education, experiences, general levels of awareness, and individual neurology. A mentally active, neurologically sound individual will evolve his or her belief system numerous times over a life span. Remaining open to the reconstruction of one's belief system is essential to individual wellbeing and to growth in social welfare.

Bell, John Stewart—Born June 28, 1928, in Belfast, Ireland, Bell was a physicist who became well known as the originator of Bell's theorem, regarded by some in the quantum mechanics community as one of the most important theorems of the twentieth century. Bell's theorem scientifically proves that in order for normal cause and effect to exist, all parts of the universe must be connected to each other instantaneously at a subatomic level, faster than the speed of light with no time lost at all (what physicists call superluminal).

Bio-electromagnetic (BioEM) energies—Field(s) of electromagnetic energy generated by the human body having characteristics similar to light. BioEM energies are understood to be a function of subtle energies generated by the human mind in the form of thought and emotion, as well as a function of activity in specific energy centers located in the spine and extremities and specific organs, such as the heart and brain.

Biophysics—A field of scientific inquiry that understands the body and biological processes using the theories and tools of physics. In particular, the understanding that the chemicals which comprise the body and all its processes are composed of atoms and subatomic energy. Willem Einthoven documented the energy field of the heart over a century ago. His research led him to invent the electrocardiogram and won him the Nobel in 1924. A quarter of a century later, Hans Berger measured the electrical fields of the brain, resulting in the discipline of electroencephalography. Biophysics provides the scientific foundation for energy medicine.

Biofield therapies—The term given to a class of energy therapies that involve strengthening, clearing, and balancing the human body's bio-electromagnetic (BioEM) energy fields as a means to heal physical, psychological, and spiritual problems.

Bohr, Niels—Born October 7, 1885, Bohr was a Danish physicist who made fundamental contributions to our understanding of atomic structure and quantum mechanics for which he received the Nobel Prize in 1922. Bohr is widely considered one of the greatest physicists of the twentieth century. He was the first to prove that electrons travel in discrete orbits around an atom's nucleus and that the the chemical properties of every element are largely determined by the number of electrons in each of these orbits. His extensive work on the Copenhagen interpretation of quantum mechanics led him to the principle of complementarity: that quantum (subatomic) energy phenomena could be analyzed separately as having several contradictory properties that operate within a single intelligent framework. His investigations led him to conclude that energy at the quantum level appears to be governed by one vast thought, expressing itself as quantum energy, which then masquerades as a complex physical universe (see *unified field theory*).

Cathartic release—In psychology, cathartic release refers to the release of stored-up or repressed emotions.

Chakra—Chakra is Sanskrit for "wheel." In Hindu and Buddhist systems of medicine, chakra refers to an energy center in the body. In both systems, major chakras are aligned in an ascending column from the base of the spine to the top of the head with numerous lesser energy centers located in other parts of the body and extremities. Each chakra is associated with specific physiological, mental, or spiritual functions. The Hindu scheme has seven major chakras. The first chakra is located at the base of the spine and is responsible for storing basic biological energy. The second chakra is located near the genitals and fuels procreative functions. The third is near the sternum, supports organ health, and serves as a location for storage of strong emotion. The fourth chakra surrounds the heart, powers the heart and lungs, and serves as a storehouse of emotions relating to love, relationships, and human virtue. The fifth charka is in the throat, powers the thyroid, and is associated with personal expression. The sixth chakra is in the forehead at the point between the eyebrows, supports neurological health, and stores the understanding of deep meaning and purpose in life. The seventh chakra is at the crown of the head, supports sophisticated brain functions, and is associated with a person's overall spiritual evolution.

Clinical psychology—The application of principles and methods from various branches of psychology as a way to study, measure, evaluate, and treat mental, behavioral, and emotional problems. The psychological science base is rich, embracing models and theories covering human sensation, perception and cognition, the neurobiological bases of behavior, thought and feeling, processes of human development, the structure of personality, the structure of human consciousness, learning processes, environmental conditioning processes, social conditioning processes, family dynamics, behavior and personality disorders, and much more. Individual psychotherapy, consisting of one-on-one verbal communication between the psychologist and the client, is the primary treatment modality used in the practice of clinical psychology, though interventions may include behavioral reeducation, environmental manipulation, group psychotherapy, couples therapy, or family therapy.

Cognition—The mental process by which a person perceives, interprets, and attributes meaning to their experiences.

Cognitive-behavioral therapy—A type of psychotherapy first developed by psychiatrist Aaron T. Beck in the 1960s. Beck concluded that the way in which his clients perceived, interpreted, and attributed meaning to their experience—a process known scientifically as cognition—was a key to therapy. Beck showed that a person's emotions and behavior result from their thought processes. He developed a list of "errors" in thinking that could cause or maintain problematic emotions and behaviors, including arbitrary inference, selective abstraction, overgeneralization, magnification of negatives, and minimization of positives. Most of the advances in the field of psychology over the last thirty years have been in the domain of cognitive-behavioral therapy. Contemporary cognitive-behavioral therapy seeks to identify and change "distorted" or "unrealistic" ways of thinking, and thereby, change emotion and behavior.

Complementary and Alternative Medicine (CAM)—A group of diverse medical and healthcare systems, practices, and products that are not currently considered to be part of conventional medicine. Examples include mind-body medicine, homeopathic medicine, naturopathic medicine, traditional Chinese medicine, herbal remedies, nutritional supplements, chiropractic and osteopathic manipulation, and biofield therapies. These interventions are considered to be complementary medicine when they are used together with conventional medicine (as when meditation is used to reduce a patient's pain following surgery). The same interventions are described as alternative medicine when they are used *in place of* conventional medicine (as when a person is using a special diet to treat cancer instead of undergoing surgery, radiation, or chemotherapy). Integrative medicine combines treatments from conventional medicine and CAM for which there is some high-quality evidence of safety and effectiveness. For more information on CAM, go to the website of the National Center for Complementary and Alternative Medicine of the National Institutes of Health at http://NCCAM.NIH.GOV.

Conscious mind—Ordinary day-to-day awareness in which an individual experiences his or herself and life in general on a "known" basis, such as the thoughts and feelings that a person is typically aware of.

Conventional medicine—Medicine as practiced by holders of medical doctor or doctor of osteopathy degrees and by health professionals such as psychologists, physical therapists, nurse practitioners, and registered nurses.

Delusion—Commonly defined as a fixed false belief, used to describe a belief that is false, fanciful, or derived from deception.

Electromagnetic fields (EMFs)—Invisible lines of electromagnetic force that permeate and surround anything through which energy flows. The earth produces EMFs, as does a thunderstorm and other electrically charged objects. The human body is also composed of energy: from the quantum energy that forms the basis for electrons, neutrons, and protons—the building blocks of chemical composition, cellular structure, and function—to the electric nerve impulses that govern the human heartbeat. EMFs in and around the human body and all organic life forms are called bio-electromagnetic energy fields (BioEM energies). Even human thought and feeling are composed of energy. When a patient is connected to an electroencephalograph (EEG), his or her brain activity is measured in the form of energy waves whose amplitude and frequency correlate with various states of consciousness (waking or sleeping, anxious or calm, for example). Likewise, energy flowing through the body creates BioEM fields whose composition, size, and fluctuation correlate with various states of physical, mental, and spiritual health. If a person's BioEM energies are strong, clear, and balanced, then his or her physical and psychological health are likely to be good, and vice versa.

Empowerment—The process of increasing the spiritual, mental, political, social, or economic strength of individuals and communities.

Energy medicine—One of four domains of Complementary and Alternative Medicine (CAM) identified by the National Center for Complementary and Alternative Medicine (NCCAM) of the National Institutes of Health, which is based on the understanding that illness results from disturbances in the body's bio-electromagnetic (BioEM) energies and that these disturbances can be addressed via electrical or electromagnetic stimulation. Many of the body's electrical systems and electromagnetic fields are well-known, well-documented, and the focus of established conventional medical interventions. The application of lasers and magnetic pulsation in specific, measurable wavelengths and frequencies have been found to be therapeutic for healing damaged tendons, repairing aneurisms, destroying cancer cells, and breaking up bone-based scar tissue.

Expressive techniques—Also referred to as "expressive therapies," the intentional use of the creative arts as a form of therapy, based on the proven assumption that creative expression, movement, and use of the imagination heal the body, mind, and spirit. Most forms of creative expression have an equivalent therapeutic discipline: art therapy, dance therapy, music therapy, drama therapy (or psychodrama), and expressive writing are examples.

Freud, Sigmund—Born May 6, 1856, Sigmund Freud was an Austrian neurologist and psychiatrist best known for his theories regarding the subconscious mind and his groundbreaking work in the field of psychoanalysis. His model of human consciousness looked like an iceberg: conscious mind is the tip of the iceberg, the part above the water while the subconscious mind (or unconscious mind) is the part of the iceberg that is hidden below the surface, many times larger and more powerful. Freud was the first to theorize that the key to mental health rests in the ability to uncover repressed memories and distorted thoughts that exist in the subconscious mind. He is often called "the father of psycho-analysis" for his pioneering work in developing the psychoanalytic method as a means to help people gain insight into their subconscious memories, emotions, and motivations. He popularized concepts like "defense mechanism," the "Freudian slip," and "dream symbolism."

Gatekeeper—In psychology, a wall that prevents the flow of knowledge, memories, or other information from one level of the mind to another. There are two gatekeepers in the mind. One gatekeeper filters content flowing between the conscious mind and the subconscious mind while the other filters content flowing between the subconscious and super-conscious minds. Hypnosis moves both gatekeepers aside by calming the mind, at which point the gatekeepers simply relax and slide out of the way, allowing access to the content of the conscious, subconscious, and super-conscious minds at the same time.

Hypnogogic state—A deep hypnotic state that naturally occurs just before falling asleep.

Hypnopompic state—A deep hypnotic state that naturally occurs just before waking up.

Hypnosis—A state of altered mental attention that can be self-induced or induced by another person (a hypnotherapist or healthcare professional trained in hypnosis). During hypnosis, a person is able to focus all his or her attention, concentrate intently on a particular subject, and experience increased knowledge about the subject, including knowledge contained in his or her subconscious and super-conscious minds. Hypnosis is a natural state of mind, common to all human beings. The trance, or focused state of mind under hypnosis, can vary from a light state to a heavy or "deep" state. A light state of hypnosis is experienced whenever a person is concentrating on something so intently that they lose awareness of their environment, as is the case when you go to your local cyber-café and sip coffee over your laptop, so engrossed in what you're doing that the noise in the café fades into the background. An example of medium hypnosis exists in the case where a consultant, whose mind is engrossed on developing a new proposal during the commute home, is unaware of the details of the drive, perhaps even unaware of having driven, right up until pulling into the driveway (called highway hypnosis). An example of deep hypnosis exists in a case where a person is induced into full anesthesia without medication, using the power of the mind to block what would otherwise be excruciating pain in a normal state of consciousness.

State-of-the-art clinical hypnosis utilizes the natural ability of the focused mind and the mind's willingness to accept positive suggestions to improve health and wellbeing. Medical research reveals a growing list of ailments that are positively affected through hypnosis when properly utilized by a trained professional for clinical purposes: (1) reducing or eliminating anxiety-related disorders, especially phobias; (2) alleviating many ailments, especially those with a psychogenic component, such as ulcers, colitis, asthma, arthritis, dysmenorrhea, fibromyalgia, and hypertension; (3) altering automatic responses to old trauma via "release" of subconscious experience of previous trauma and restructuring subconscious reaction to further "cues" of trauma; (4) eliminating unhealthy habits, such as smoking and overeating; (5) alleviating chronic pain and achieving full anesthesia, as in the case of painless childbirth; (6) improving clinical outcomes related to medical and dental procedures; and (7) enhancing learning, from improved memorization to receiving and understanding complex insights regarding physical, psychological, and spiritual issues.

Hypnotic guided imagery—Use of imagery to guide an individual into a hypnotic state, deepen the hypnotic trance state, and aid in accomplishing specific goals for healing during hypnosis. Use of guided imagery during a hypnotic induction helps the subject (person being hypnotized) move attention away from the outside world and toward a relaxed and focused inner awareness. It can be used to deepen a person's trance state and to heighten bodily awareness under hypnosis and is therefore integral to hypnotic processes, which are focused on reducing physical and mental stress, healing illness or injury, inducing pain relief (analgesia), or full body anesthesia. Guided imagery is also used effectively to help achieve specialized goals under hypnosis, such as weight loss, smoking cessation, and behavior modification.

Hypnotic induction—A formalized group of words, phrases, and images that move a subject's attention away from the outside world and toward a relaxed and focused inner awareness (a hypnotic state). There are many different types of inductions. Certain inductions work better for particular personality types. Inductions also vary depending on the desired depth of the trance state and the type of work to be accomplished while the subject is under hypnosis. A simple induction has three parts. The first part is a basic focusing and relaxing proce-dure, often a ten-to-one countdown using a variety of voice modulations and prompts. The second part is a bodily relaxation procedure, often a progressive relaxation method using direct suggestion. The third part involves deepening the trance state, often through the use of hypnotic guided imagery.

Integrative medicine—The term used to describe the combined use of con-ventional medicine with complementary and alternative medicine (CAM) for which there is some rigorous research-based evidence of safety and effective-ness. An example would be using meditation following heart surgery to reduce pain, expedite post-surgical recovery, manage stress, and help maintain contin-ued heart health.

Intuition—A form of ready, accurate insight that arises independent of a per-son's previous experiences or empirical knowledge.

Jung, Carl—Born July 26, 1875, Carl Gustav Jung was a Swiss psychiatrist, a colleague of Sigmund Freud, and founder of analytical psychology. His broad and unique approach to psychology included the application of a rigorous sci-entific method but also emphasized understanding the mind through exploring the worlds of religion, philosophy, mythology, and symbolism. Jung's work focused heavily on the "unconscious," which would include the subconscious as Freud defined it, plus what Jung called "the collective unconscious," a store-house of latent memory traces inherited from man's ancestral past, including not only the history of man as a separate species but our pre-human ancestry as well, the whole history of human evolution. Jung discovered that this collective unconscious is shared by all people and is therefore universal, and he under-stood it to be the foundation upon which the individual subconscious mind and ego are built. According to Jung, included in the collective unconscious are "archetypes," basic human personality patterns that we live out from deep inside ourselves and the collective culture.

Kabat-Zinn, Jon—Associate Professor of Medicine at the University of Massa-chusetts Medical School, Dr. Kabat-Zinn has conducted numerous studies and published several books that focus on mind-body interventions that promote healing. His Mindfulness-Based Stress Reduction (MBSR) program, an eight-week course that combines meditation and hatha yoga, has been demonstrated to effect positive changes in brain activity, stress reduction, improved emotional processing, better immune functioning, and symptom amelioration in people who suffer from chronic pain, stress-related illnesses, and/or a wide range of chronic diseases, including breast cancer. Over 200 medical centers and clinics nationwide and abroad now use the MBSR model. Dr. Kabat-Zinn received his PhD in molecular biology in 1971 from MIT.

Magnetic pull—A process that occurs naturally during the use of any scientifically based meditation technique, during which neurological energy is withdrawn from the peripheral nervous system, concentrated in the spine, and then channeled upward to the brain. The practical result of magnetic pull during meditation is that the meditator experiences a withdrawal of sensory awareness from the outside world (because there is less energy in the peripheral nervous system), is thereby able to limit sensory distractions to achieve a calm, inward focus, and has more energy available to support mental and spiritual functions.

Meditation—Methods for calming and focusing the mind. Meditation is the mental "laboratory work" through which people come to master their own mental and physical states and achieve the expansion of conscious awareness. There are many secularized forms of meditation that are effectively used in contemporary society for therapy and relaxation. Recognizing the need for meditative practice in the stress and strain of modern life, secular psychology has produced a variety of therapies (Gestalt Therapy, for example) that represent secularized versions of classical religious meditative disciplines. For example, certain forms of humanistic and transpersonal psychology have championed the expansion of human potential through meditative techniques, such as biofeedback. Dr. Jon Kabat-Zinn and other researchers in the health sciences have identified a number of therapeutic benefits derived from meditation, including: (1) improved rates of recovery from a variety of illnesses, especially those with a psychogenic component, such as such as ulcers, asthma, arthritis, fibromyalgia, and hypertension; (2) improved circulation, vitality, and stamina; (3) management of chronic pain; (4) improved clinical outcomes associated with dental and medical treatments; (5) reduced anxiety, fear, and depression; (6) greater mental clarity and peace of mind; and (7) experience of insights relating to one's social, psychological, and physical wellbeing, as well as answers to questions regarding the meaning and purpose of life.

There are many schools of meditative practice, with the following approaches common: (1) body preparation via progressive relaxation, yoga, Tai Chi, and so forth; (2) specific postures; (3) set opening phrases or patterns of prayer; (4) chant; (5) concentration on single word mantras, sounds, or repetitive phrases; (6) use of the breath and breathing to calm the mind and focus attention; (7) methods of mindfulness designed to erase "mental static" created by intruding thoughts and feelings; (8) means for withdrawing attention from the senses and all external stimuli; and (9) methods for achieving one-pointed concentration on the object of one's meditation, whether it be improved health, greater mental clarity and peace, or God.

Contemporary meditative methods evolved mostly from ancient religious sources. Hinduism, Taoism, Buddhism, Judaism, Sufism, Sikhism, Christianity, and other spiritual traditions have long utilized meditation to expand the human consciousness in order to achieve the unifying of an individual's life and being with ultimate, Universal Truth. Spiritual meditation equates to mastering and focusing the mind to achieve perfect concentration on God, Tao, Brahman, Nirvana, Jehovah, or Allah, depending on religious perspective. Spiritual meditation is understood to depend for its result on the action of God's grace (the Western perspective) or on the essential unity between the individual human soul and the Universal Soul of God (the Eastern perspective).

Medulla oblongata—The brain stem, located at the base of the brain. This part of the brain directly controls breathing, blood flow, heartbeat, and many other essential functions. In Eastern medicine, specifically Hindu and Buddhist medicine, this area coincides with an important energy center—the medullary center—through which energy flows into the body.

Mind-body medicine—Techniques designed to enhance the mind's capacity to affect bodily function and health. Mind-body medicine focuses on the interactions among the brain, mind, body, and behavior and the ways in which emotional, mental, social, spiritual, and behavioral factors directly impact physical health and wellbeing. Mind-body intervention strategies that are thought to promote health include hypnosis, meditation, yoga, cognitive-behavioral therapies, Tai Chi, group support, autogenic training, and spirituality. Some mind-body approaches have been documented to be effective and are considered mainstream, such as cognitive therapy, hypnosis, meditation, and expressive therapies. Other mind-body techniques, such as prayer, though widely considered effective, are still being researched for their effectiveness.

Neuroscience—The scientific study concerned with the structure, function, development, genetics, biochemistry, physiology, pharmacology, and pathology of the central and peripheral nervous systems. Neuroscience focuses chiefly on an investigation of the brain and central nervous systems, with special focus on how people perceive and interact with the external world and how human experience and biology influence each other. The scope of neuroscience has become very broad over the last two decades, signaling a convergence of interest in the fields of psychology, computer science, statistics, physics, medicine, sociology, and economics. There are several subspecialties within the field of neuroscience. Cognitive neuroscience addresses how psychological and cognitive functions are produced by neural circuitry, and vice versa. Social neuroscience focuses on the brain's interaction with the environment. Neurobiology is sometimes confused with neuroscience. The former term refers to the biology of the nervous system and the latter term refers to the science of neural circuitries and their relationship to mental and physical functions in the human body and the surrounding environment.

Philosophy—A discipline concerned with the critical examination of the rational grounds for our most fundamental beliefs and logical analysis of the basic concepts employed in the expression of such beliefs. Philosophy is perhaps the oldest and most highly regarded of the sciences. It has been a recognized discipline since the days of the ancient Greek philosophers and has evolved over more than 2,500 years based on the questions that have been relevant to society at any given point. What were once purely philosophical pursuits have evolved into the modern specialized fields of psychology, sociology, linguistics, and economics. Philosophical rigor informs all modern sciences, medicine, mathematics, politics, and linguistics. There are four main branches of philosophy: ethics (moral conduct with respect to rightness or wrongness), metaphysics (the essential nature of things), epistemology (what counts as genuine knowledge), and logic (the correct principles of reasoning). Each branch has several sub-classifications. For example, within metaphysics, ontology is the inquiry into the meaning of existence itself, and philosophy of mind is an inquiry into the nature of the mind, consciousness (awareness), mental functions and properties, and their relationship to the physical body. The vast body of philosophy is divided into historical periods and classified by particular schools of thought. A complete survey of philosophy is unfortunately beyond the scope of this summary.

Pro re nata (PRN)—A Latin term literally meaning "for the thing born" but used in medicine to mean "as needed." Most often used in the administration of medication when a patient or caregiver is allowed to administer doses of medication outside of prescribed levels on an as-needed basis.

Progressive relaxation (PR)—In hypnosis, refers to progressive relaxation of the body using one or more methods: a ten-to-one countdown, direct suggestion, focused breathing, guided imagery, or progressive tensing and relaxing of muscle groups. Progressive relaxation techniques are often utilized as part of a hypnotic induction but may be used at any time during hypnosis to promote further relaxation and deepen the trance state. Outside of hypnosis, PR techniques can be self-induced or utilized with the guidance of another person, such as a psychologist, social worker, or physical therapist. They reduce stress, anxiety, and physiological tension in the body and have the added benefits of lowering pulse rate and blood pressure.

Psychogenic—In medicine, of mental or emotional origin. Refers most often to the psychological stimulus for disease or illness in the body. Certain illnesses, such as asthma, arthritis, fibromyalgia, heart disease, hypertension, and ulcers, are considered to have a strong psychogenic (mental) component. Severe stress, depression, anxiety, grief, or trauma are known psychogenic factors that contribute to the onset and severity of physical illness. Psychogenic illness is not to be confused with psychosomatic illness, which is the artificial creation of symptoms caused by mental processes of the sufferer without physiological cause. With psychogenic illness, the illness also has a biological basis; it is real.

Psychotherapy—An interpersonal, relational intervention used by trained psychotherapists to help clients deal with a wide range of mental and emotional problems. Typically, therapy takes on the overall focus of increasing one's sense of wellbeing and reducing subjective discomforting experiences and thoughts. There are a wide range of techniques used in psychotherapy based on experiential relationship building, dialogue, communication, and behavior change. These techniques are designed to improve the mental health of a client or to improve relationships, such as in a couple or family. Most forms of psychotherapy employ the use of spoken conversation (talk therapy) with the inclusion of specific therapeutic techniques. Some forms also use various other techniques of communication, such as the written word, psychodrama, or other expressive techniques. Psychotherapy occurs within a structured encounter between a trained therapist and client(s). Therapy is generally used to respond to a variety of specific or nonspecific manifestations of clinically diagnosable problems or crises. Treatment of everyday problems, by contrast, is often referred to as "counseling" though this term is often used interchangeably with "psychotherapy."

Quantum mechanics—The branch of physics that deals with how energy behaves at the atomic and subatomic levels. The term derives from the Latin word quantum, meaning "how much." Quanta are the discrete subatomic energy packets that are the building blocks of light waves. Accepted theories of quantum mechanics were established during the first half of the twentieth century by Max Planck, Werner Heisenberg, Niels Bohr, Erwin Schrödinger, and others who wanted to explain the behaviors and characteristics of quantum energy (light at the atomic and subatomic levels), which behaves in ways that cannot be explained by classic Newtonian physics, classic theories of electromagnetism, or Albert Einstein's general theory of relativity. Quantum mechanics led to a number of accepted and important theories. Planck's quantum hypothesis explained how the energy radiated by an atomic system is proportional to the radiant energy generated by each discrete energy element in the system. Werner Heisenberg's uncertainty principle resolved what had been a major quandry regarding the inability to precisely locate electrons in an atomic unit. Einstein built upon Planck's work to show that an electromagnetic wave, such as light, also consists of tiny energy particles called photons. This led to the theory of wave-particle duality, in which particles and waves were neither one nor the other but had certain properties of both. While quantum mechanics describes the world of the very small, it also helps explain how certain "macroscopic" quantum systems behave, such as superconductors. Quantum mechanics is regarded widely by professional physicists as the most fundamental framework we have for understanding and describing nature.

Quantum super-position—An established characteristic of electromagnetic energy fields at the quantum level. Every organism, place, and thing in existence possesses its own electromagnetic energy field(s). At the quantum (subatomic) level, these fields generate energy waves with the potential for a wide range of tendencies or possibilities. The wave-particle duality theory of quantum mechanics shows that when two fields interact, they formulate energy particles that transfer momentum and energy between the two fields. Simply put, the energy fields between two objects emit and absorb exchanged particles, in effect playing a subatomic game of "catch" at the point they encounter one another. When that happens, the undifferentiated waves of energy contained in both fields are altered, discrete energy particles are created, and a specific outcome—one of many possible tendencies that existed in the original energy waves of both objects—will occur.

Religion—Religion has so many meanings that it is almost ill-advised to capture its essence in a single definition. The following description is drawn in part from *The Encyclopedia of Religion*: a push toward ultimacy, deepest truth, and transcendence that provides norms and power for living. When distinct patterns of behavior, a shared history, codified doctrines, rituals, and sacraments are built around this type of depth dimension, the resulting structure consitutes "religion" in a recognizable form. Organized religion generally refers to an organization of people who share a prescribed set of beliefs, ethical standards, and rituals, usually taking the form of a legal entity. The term religion is sometimes used interchangeably with faith or spirituality, but these latter terms are more closely associated with personal conviction or a personal belief in the sacred or holy, not necessarily associated with organized religion.

Repetition compulsion—A repetitive pattern of flawed thought, feeling, and/or behavior that has dire consequences for health and wellbeing. Unresolved difficult experiences or emotions create impressions in the subconscious mind that lead to repetitive, negative tendencies of thought, feeling, and behavior. People who suffer from repetition compulsions are prone to react in a specific way to a particular situation or stimulus, even when their response is harmful. One example consists of a woman raised by an emotionally distant father, who in adulthood repeatedly pursues intimate relationships with men who are emotionally unavailable like her father.

Repression—The psychological act of excluding feelings, thoughts, fantasies, or desires from one's conscious awareness and attempting to hold or subdue them in the subconscious. Repression is usually an unconscious mechanism (we do it without being aware of it) that can be detrimental to mental and physical health. People tend to repress an experience they find painful, terrifying, difficult, shameful, or otherwise challenging. We often dismiss or deny painful emotions as a means to maintain psychological stability, or because we simply don't have time to deal with them in the face of our responsibilities. Unfortunately, powerful feelings, thoughts, and desires that are repressed in this manner remain in the subconscious mind, where they sabotage our psychological, spiritual, and physical wellbeing (see *psychogenic illness*). Repressed emotion can be safely released through psychotherapy, hypnosis, expressive techniques, and other tools of contemporary psychology. Repression is not the same as thought suppression, which is entirely conscious, and thus, can be more readily dealt with.

Stress—A response of the sympathetic nervous system that arises when there is an unacceptable disparity between your expectations/needs and what you actually experience. Stress activates the sympathetic leg of the nervous system and the release of stress hormones that amp up production of adrenaline and divert blood flow to the large muscles. The body needs this power because it "thinks" it has to run away from or fight something. This is the so-called fight or flight response. When you are in this response mode, blood flows more to the heart and large muscles and correspondingly less to the digestive system and other vital organs that are not immediately necessary for a fight or flight. The immediate effects are dry mouth, motor agitation, sweating, heart palpitations, increased blood pressure, enlarged pupils, sleeplessness, and mental anxiety.

There is such a thing as good stress. The challenges posed in our lives have the potential to enhance our physical and mental functioning. However, if stress is chronic and excessive, it eventually causes harm. Chronic stress can cause anger or rage, fear or terror, fragmented or distorted thinking, impatience, emotional lability (erratic emotional states), memory loss, anxiety, and depression. Stress is closely associated with hypertension, heart disease, stroke, arthritis, gastro-intestinal disorders, and other health problems. According to the American Academy of Family Physicians, two-thirds of office visits to family doctors are for stress-related symptoms.

Subconscious mind—An aspect of the mind that operates outside of ordinary conscious awareness but exerts tremendous influence on how we feel, think, perceive, and behave. The subconscious mind is a hidden storehouse of memory, deep feeling, desires, motives, thought, and other aspects of mind with which most people are not aware. It contains a catalogue of one's life experiences, along with the thoughts and feelings associated with important events in the past, all of which are stored in the form of subtle impressions in the subconscious mind. When, in the course of day-to-day experience, specific conditions arise that "cue" the content of the subconscious, these subtle impressions can surface into conscious awareness. The subconscious also comes to the fore any time people do something by rote memory, such as brushing teeth or driving a car—things people do "without even thinking about them," in which case, the subconscious mind is doing their thinking for them. In psychology, certain forms of psychotherapy (the psychoanalytic method in particular) and hypnosis are used to access the content of the subconscious mind, often for the purpose of releasing repressed emotional pain and distorted thought. Within the field of psychology, Sigmund Freud and Carl Jung were early pioneers who developed models for understanding the subconscious mind (also referred to in the literature as the unconscious, though the unconscious and subconscious minds are not the same).

Super-conscious awareness—A state of mind characterized by greatly reduced external awareness and expanded interior awareness which is frequently accompanied by penetrating intuitive insight, emotional (and sometimes physical) euphoria, and occasionally, visions. Although the experience is usually brief in physical time, such experiences can last several days or more, recur with frequency, and be maintained with constancy in the spiritually advanced person. Subjective perception of time, space, and/or self may strongly change during this state of consciousness. The euphoria experienced in this state of mind, sometimes described as a state of ever-new joy, is referred to as "bliss" (the Eastern religious model) or "ecstacy" (the Western religious model).

Super-conscious mind—Levels of mind, existing in every human being, that are infinite in power and capacity. There are two levels to the super-conscious mind: individual super-conscious mind and universal super-consciousness. Individual super-conscious mind is a level of "thought" or consciousness that is capable of sensing and influencing electromagnetic energy fields. Using this level of thought, we have the power to control our own personal electromagnetic energy fields (BioEM energies), as well as the electromagnetic energy fields associated with other people, places, and things. People of faith refer to this level of mind as "soul" or "spirit." The form of thought that is required to access the individual super-conscious mind is intuitive thought, which is a deep, immediate, and accurate sense of knowing something that could not necessarily be known through simple logic. The intuitive thought of individual super-conscious mind is a gateway to an even larger field of intelligent energy, the universal super-conscious mind—a single mammoth conscious energy field that exists back behind the near infinite number of individual electromagnetic energy fields that make up the entire universe. This reality is sometimes referred to in physics as the unified field—a single quantum (or subatomic) field that behaves in predictable, elegant, intelligent ways to create, sustain, and explain the structure of the universe. Within this field, everything in the universe is instantaneously connected to and reacting with everything else. People of faith refer to universal super-conscious mind as God, Jehovah, Adonai, Tao, Nirvana, Sat, Brahma, or other terms, depending upon religious perspective. Both the scientific humanist and the person of deep faith access universal super-conscious awareness via meditative thought.

Unified field—In physics, understood to be a single field of energy whose characteristics can explain and unify all four existing physical forces described below, which at present do not appear to operate according to the same principles. Continued to be highly sought after by physicists, the unified field theory aims to reconcile the four fundamental forces (energy fields) in nature: (1) strong nuclear force, the force responsible for holding quarks together to form neutrons and protons, and holding neutrons and protons together to form nuclei; (2) electromagnetic force, the familiar force that acts on electrically charged particles; (3) weak nuclear force, responsible for radioactivity; and (4) gravitational force, a long-range force of attraction that acts on all particles with mass. Notable physicists have been pursuing a unified field theory since the early 1800s and many important discoveries have resulted from their efforts. However, they have yet to formulate a consistent theory that combines general relativity and quantum mechanics. In recent years, the quest for a unified field has largely focused on string theory and its derivatives, M-theory for example. The unified field theory is sometimes confused with the Theory of Everything, which attempts to explain all four fundamental forces in nature together with the theory of general relativity *and* the nature of elementary particles that form matter.

Yoga—Sanskrit for "union," refers to one of the six schools of Hindu philosophy that describes the path to enlightenment (or knowledge of God). Hindu texts establishing the basis for yoga include the Upanishads, the Bhagavad-Gita, the Yoga Sutras of Patanjali, the Hatha Yoga Pradipika, and many others. In India, yoga is seen as a means to both physiological and spiritual mastery. Since the *Bhagavad-Gita* was written, the main branches of yoga have been classified as Hatha Yoga, attaining enlightenment through asanas (postures) and breath control; Karma Yoga, attaining enlightenment through good works; Jnana Yoga, attaining enlightenment through wisdom; Bhakti Yoga, attaining enlightenment through devotion; and Raja Yoga, attaining enlightenment through a balanced spiritual life that has meditation as its hub. Outside India, Yoga has become primarily associated with Hatha Yoga, though Raja Yoga has been popularized in the West by Paramahansa Yogananda.

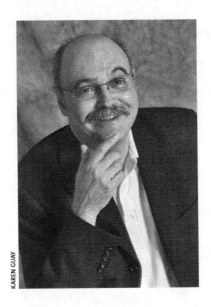

KAREN GUAY

Rick Levy, PhD, a clinician, board-certified doctor of psychology, and researcher, has been working at the forefront of mind-body medicine since 1976. A licensed psychologist in private practice, serving an international clientele, Dr. Levy has taken his techniques to five continents, to people of every culture, class, and age, from the world's international power elite to the indigenous peoples of the Amazon and Africa. He has used his methods to help in the healing of people with everything from lower back pain to lifethreatening disease. Levy's work has been featured on *Prime Time Live*, *FOX News*, PBS, and ABC radio, and in *The Washingtonian* and *The Washington Post*. He lives in Gaithersburg, Maryland, where he directs his clinic, The Levy Center for the Healing Arts.

Lou Aronica is the author of several works of fiction and nonfiction. He has collaborated on a number of books, including the national bestseller *The Culture Code*. Prior to that, he spent two decades as a senior executive in the publishing industry. He lives with his family in southern Connecticut.

Printed in the United States
by Baker & Taylor Publisher Services